Two Cookies & A Mile

Two Cookies & A Mile

Your guide to getting the most out of the
good life.

Gary L. Hansel
Edited by Matt Bourjaily

Writers Club Press
San Jose New York Lincoln Shanghai

Two Cookies & A Mile

Your guide to getting the most out of the good life.

Writers Club Press
an imprint of iUniverse, Inc.

For information address:
iUniverse, Inc.
5220 S. 16th St., Suite 200
Lincoln, NE 68512
www.iuniverse.com

ISBN: 0-595-23396-1

Printed in the United States of America

The journey only has meaning with love. My twin daughters, Stacey Jones and Jenifer Hansel, who are eleven years apart in age, and my new wife, Nancy Lyon, prove it.

Contents

Foreword ix

Author's Note xi

CHAPTER 1   Introduction, or, Please, Please Read This
First. 1

CHAPTER 2   Fat Begets Fat...and Hypertension, Diabetes,
Cancer, Strokes, Heart Attacks, and On and
On, and Worse 15

CHAPTER 3   Eat Less & Less, Weigh More & More. In
Other Words, Diets Don't Work 21

CHAPTER 4   Masticating Correctly...and Ole' Olestra 27

CHAPTER 5   Calories Don't Count. No, Calories Do Count.
Wait. What I Really Want To Say Is: Yes,
Overweight People Often Eat Less Than Thin
People 45

CHAPTER 6   Metabolism: The Slow & The Fast, and It
Doesn't Matter 49

CHAPTER 7   Exercise, Lexercise, and Butt-Sitting 55

CHAPTER 8   Stretching 77

CHAPTER 9   Ladies, Please. 79

CHAPTER 10   Why Do Overweight People Lift Weights To
Lose Weight? 83

CHAPTER 11   Pretty Pink Bra...i.e., Get Some Support 85

CHAPTER 12   "Doc, It Hurts When I Do This." "Then Don't
Do That." or, The Irresponsibility of the
Medical Community and Other Credentialed
People and Organizations 89

CHAPTER 13   Excuses, Excuses, and More Excuses 93

CHAPTER 14   "It's In My Genes." "No, It's In Your
Jeans.". 95

CHAPTER 15   Stress (Chill Out. Relax. Life Is Real Short,
Right Suzie?). 99

CHAPTER 16   Willpower, Discipline, Motivation and
SEX 103

CHAPTER 17   Drugs, Pills, Herbals, Miracles, Natural
Remedies, Vitamins, Minerals, Supplements,
Zen-Zen, I Mean Fen-Phen, And Other
Stupid Things. 107

CHAPTER 18   Ageless Wonders: For the Old, Older, and
Oldest. 117

CHAPTER 19   Kids Are Cute...and Fat and Getting Fatter
All the Time 123

CHAPTER 20   The Author and the DeSoto 125

Foreword

I am just trying to help people, but I am being selfish, too. I want to enjoy life and make each day special, fulfilling, and fun. Like most of us talk about doing, but don't do very often. There aren't many days when we actually pull it off, because real life keeps getting in the way.

I have learned that when I try to help others with something, I wind up helping myself. Like trying to experience the good in life. In working with others to do that, I get more out of life myself. I stay healthy, fit, and thin, my mind operates in a sharper manner, and I enjoy the day.

The point is, I am in this with you. I have tried to do in this book for the reader what I would do for myself, which is to make things as easy and clear as possible. I hope you will read along comfortably, and that you will benefit from whatever this book might offer.

Let's enjoy the day.

Author's Note

I much prefer information that is short and to the point. Unfortunately, most information comes in the opposite form, and this is especially true in the areas of health, fitness, and weight loss. In these areas, there is an inordinate amount of information, and far too much of it is bad, making it difficult to learn.

It is my purpose to help people, so in this book I have endeavored to provide good information that is easy to read, understand, and use. I hope the reader finds it clear and helpful.

I wish everyone well, and I sincerely encourage input. Please feel free to track me down via **www.garylhansel.com**

1

Introduction, or, Please, Please Read This First

It's been great, the good life. We've had it all: education, careers, money, houses, cars, and more. But the good life has presented us with threats to the enjoyment of our success, in spite of what knowledge and action should have prevented. But what the heck, we can do anything, as we have proven, so we can deal with this, too.

I am a "half-full" person, and accordingly, I look at this situation and kind of grin. Not at the potential problems, but at the way they came about. There we were, moving along and jazzing around, accomplishing things that were unheard of not all that long ago, doing whatever we wanted, and conquering everything in our path. But we forgot to take care of ourselves along the way. Like planning a trip by car, packing, and driving to where we intended to go, only to get out of the car when we arrived and discovering the baby on the roof. It seems we sat that sweet girl there in her car seat and forgot to move her into the car before we took off. We forgot to take care of something very important. The good news is the baby is still there, had a great ride, and is now looking forward to a nice meal of mashed-up bananas. Like us making the trip along the good life's highway only to discover that we forgot about our health and well-being. And suddenly, but not too late, realizing that even though our cholesterol was elevated, our arteries had begun to get a bit clogged up, and we were overweight, we had time to fix it all. Wonderful. Now we do our thing and properly analyze the situation and solve the problems. So, here we go. Just in time too, because we could be just two more cookies away from real trouble, and if we tried to run off those cookies, we wouldn't be able to. Our poor eating habits and lack of exercise have taken their tolls.

The good news for us is that we have the talents and can-do attitudes to fix these things. That is why I call this a happy book. We can enjoy our success by reversing some of the problems the good life has created. Before we move on, though, let me ask that you remain open-minded for a while, because you might read some things that go against the grain. Let's at least get through the bulk of the material before anyone starts slinging anything, because once we get into things a ways, they should begin to add up. (If they don't, at least I will know when to duck.)

This Is All About Good Things

This book is about living life with health, vigor, and enthusiasm. About having fun and enjoying the day. It revolves around positive things and reflects what I believe people want. Since we have earned the opportunity to enjoy life, we should take it upon ourselves to see that we get as much out of it as possible.

There is just so much good to experience, and I am offering help to those who would agree. This book really isn't meant to be any more than that. Just good news about how to put ourselves in position to enjoy the good life. Along this line, it is not my intent to convince anyone that they have a problem, but rather to offer input to those who have at least some awareness of the situation and are concerned about fixing things. This book will add a sense of urgency, though, regarding solution, because I believe so strongly in the possibilities for growth and happiness. Space is used, then, to define and clarify the issues to help people's understanding in the hope that doing so will make it easier for them to get going. Now let's get going.

Setting Things Up

A little history and philosophy might be good here, at this early stage of the book, to contribute to whatever value I have to offer the reader. Both in the Author's Note and the Foreword, I have stated that all I am trying to do is help, and that is all there is to this. Much flows from that, though, such as the following:

A. A lot will be written condemning magic and miracles and other such impossible remedies, and be assured that none of those types of expectations are raised in this book. It is not possible to help people while at the same time creating hope for quick fixes with no effort. This book is all about eating right and exercising. Nothing else. I bring this up early, so that a reader will not be hurriedly flipping through the pages in search of the "sorcerer's stone." (I just finished reading the first Harry Potter book.)

B. My credentials for writing this book might be challenged at first glance, but after you see the following, a different perspective should arise:

> The problems are vast in terms of scope, magnitude, and severity.

> Americans spend tens of billions of dollars annually trying to make things better while things keep getting worse.

> Most all of the advice people follow while attempting to fix things comes from professionals formally trained in health, fitness, and weight

With the above in mind, you could (and as far as I am concerned, should) conclude that the credentialed people might be (or must be) wrong. I drew that conclusion, because it is painted thick all over society. The problems are obvious, and as far as I am concerned, so are the solutions. It is possible that since I am not a formally trained nutritionist, medical person, exercise instructor or whatever, that I am able to try and help people become healthy, fit, and thin without the blinders that the formally trained must have been fitted for in school. Strong words, I know. But if (for example) dieting actually causes weight gain over time (and this book hopes to show that it does), and excess weight often leads to other problems such as heart disease, high blood pressure, and more, and the formally trained continue to advise people to go on diets, then the formally trained are wrong. I cannot draw any other conclusion, especially when everything I have seen and researched points to the same thing: in the long run eating right and exercise always work while dieting fails nearly 100% of the time and actually makes things worse nearly 100% of the time.

So here I am, and here is the book, and please give both a chance. If there is no magic and the credentialed have failed, what can be wrong with trying the tried and true?

C. The tried and true have been lost in the shuffle of the good times. That is why I am going down the road of back-to-basics. It seems that in the quest for miracles the keys to the underlying things that work have been misplaced. For example, a person might go to the grocery store and walk out with a bit of wholesome, healthy food in one hand and high-fat ice cream in the other with the erroneous thought that all is well. Such a person might think that switching part of the bad food to good will offset all the bad, when in reality the bad is so bad, nothing good will come of such partial efforts. It is our dramatically poor eating habits that have caused our problems, and the facts to support that are clear in the literature but fuzzy in the mind. Therefore, a refocus is essential. This book attempts to clear things up, at least enough to where meaningful change has a chance to take place, because change is what is needed and wanted by so many, as evidenced by the enormous amounts of money spent on fake remedies.

If those things that have been done on the advice of the formally trained have not only not worked but have actually made things worse, a search in another direction has to be undertaken.

Now to the Toll

Don't be alarmed. Just look at what has taken place while we were shaking up the world. I will be as gentle as possible.

As Newsweek magazine points out (8-2-99), "…our way of life fosters an array of deadly ills, from hypertension and heart disease to diabetes and some cancers…[and] we've hardly begun to confront what is happening to us."

And it all keeps getting worse, as evidenced by the fact that Americans spend tens of billions of dollars a year on various health, fitness, and weight loss plans, scams and schemes, and they get heavier, more unhealthy, and more unfit with every passing year. As shown in a 5-29-99 Chicago Tribune article, obesity costs more than $70 billion annually in direct healthcare expenses or in lost productivity. Other lifestyle-caused problems aren't even in these figures.

We have been ruining our health, getting heavier, and worse. All the money and success we have earned will not help. Knowledge and action will. As a Harvard University School of Public Health study found, "…unhealthy habits and an unhealthy lifestyle cause 65 percent of cancer deaths." Unbelievable, but hardly surprising, because we refuse to acknowledge reality, while we embrace the ridiculous. The reality is that (1) we have widespread lifestyle-caused problems, and (2) rather than take responsibility by utilizing our vast knowledge and American problem-solving abilities to fix things, we (3) rely on hocus-pocus, miracles, and other such remedies that often make things worse.

This is ridiculous. Let's fix things. This is where the "happy book" statement of earlier comes in, because solving problems can be fun. Since we have spent such an enormous amount of time, effort, and money only to make things worse, we can smile as we move on to the happier days that will follow as we become healthy, fit, and thin. When we begin doing this, we will be able to maximize our mental and physical capabilities and be much better able to enjoy our futures. And the future starts now.

NOTE

In order to make things better, we need to be realistic while discarding myth and the ridiculous. So here are a few thoughts to set the stage for what follows throughout this book:

1. Most people, by the time they hit their late 20's, have all three of the following:

> Elevated cholesterol

> Partially clogged arteries

> Excess weight

The fact that most people deny or ignore some or all of their excess weight and don't know their cholesterol is elevated and their arteries are partially clogged does not eliminate the truth. So, face the facts, check if you don't know, note the information, and begin dealing with things in an active manner.

2. The health and weight problems are closely related, because they come from the same place. Since the weight issue is much better known and more visible, this book will focus on weight as the avenue to address all the problems. As a person begins doing the things that are necessary to lose weight, other positive changes will also start to occur. This book, then, is not a diet book; it is a live well book.

3. A person starting out thin in their youth will remain thin by eating right. That person does not need to exercise to stay thin. Eating correctly will do it. However, since this book is about the total of being healthy, fit, and thin, that person will want to exercise to obtain as many of the benefits of exercise as possible.

The point here is that there is too much given to the idea that people are overweight because of a lack of exercise. While I am a huge supporter of exercise, have been exercising for thirty-two years, and couldn't imagine life without exercise, I am only making the point that it is our lousy eating habits that have caused most of our problems. We need to know this, or we will not be able to fix things. If a person eats correctly it is impossible to be overweight, as will be seen later in the chapter on eating properly (Chapter 4, Masticating Correctly…and Ole' Olestra).

4. If a person who has eaten terribly their whole live has been exercising (and this is rare), they would most likely still be overweight. They might not be as overweight as if they didn't exercise, and in even rarer circumstances such a person might actually be thin, but in either case, two facts remain:

> First: There is no amount of exercise that will produce good health if lousy eating habits exist.

> Second: Even if a person ate badly but managed to exercise enough to be at a normal, thin weight (which again is nearly impossible), that person would still have high cholesterol and partially clogged arteries, and, therefore, would still be at risk for many lifestyle-caused illnesses and diseases.

It's the food. Eating correctly is an absolute.

5. If a person eats badly all their life and never exercises, (which is most everyone), and as a result becomes unfit, unhealthy, and overweight, with elevated cholesterol and partially clogged arteries, that person can only reverse those problems by eating right and exercising. There is no other way. There are no drugs, herbs, or magic that will transform a person into being healthy, fit, and thin. While it was noted above that a lack of exercise has not been a primary cause of excess weight, exercise is a must for getting rid of the extra weight and for reversing the problems our lifestyle has cre-

ated. For those who might be thinking that exercise is impossible, that they will never be able to exercise no matter how much they want to, this book will show a way that will work for them and for anyone.

Now, let's smile, have fun, and get on with it. Then we can eat those extra two cookies. But first:

The Road Map Story

We have been deluged for years with bad information in the areas of health, fitness, and weight loss, and we believe far too much of it. Would you believe the following could happen? I do.

There was a wonderful, intelligent, successful, educated, woman named Sally, (fine looking too) living in Chicago. She wanted to drive to the west coast, so she went to a widely advertised authority on driving directions and got a map. With the great map in hand she left Chicago, dreaming about the things she was going to do when she got to the west coast. Two days later she drove up to the ocean…on the east coast. The Atlantic Ocean, not the Pacific. She meant to go west, she had gotten a map by an expert that directed her to go west, but she wound up east. Completely opposite.

Disappointed, Sally returned to Chicago, found a different expert on driving directions and headed out again. Two days later, she pulled up, again, to the east coast instead of the west coast. By this time she is mad, sad, confused, and anxious. Getting to the west coast was important to her. She had family out there she hadn't seen in years, old study buddies she hadn't been with since college, and she had an interview scheduled for a fantastic new job. Not only was a great time in store for her as she drove up and down the west coast seeing all those people, but her future looked bright as well. And she couldn't get there. Back to Chicago, to another map person, and back to the east coast instead of the west coast. She continued this forever. Her relatives disowned her, because she never showed up, her college buddies wrote her off, and the big time, big bucks job was given to someone less qualified than Sally.

Sally's deal is not as silly as it seems, because that is exactly what people do who want to lose weight and become healthy, fit, and thin. They go with directions from a weight loss expert, lose weight, then gain back whatever weight was lost plus a few more pounds. They then go to a different weight loss expert, attempt that regiment (or diet), lose weight, then gain back all that lost weight plus more, then on the next plan. After each such experience, this person weighs more than at the conclusion of the last, so that over time, the person gets heavier and heavier. Since we know that excess weight can lead to illness and disease, this person doesn't just get heavier, he or she also gets more unhealthy. And so it goes. It is as ridiculous as the trip Sally attempted. It seems that there is never a point where people say, "Wait. This isn't working. In fact, what I have been doing has not only not fixed things, they have actually made things worse. I better stop this craziness and get the right directions."

Now a few notes on the road map story:

1. I used a female, Sally, not because I am sexist, but because it is women who spend the majority of time, effort, and money on the various health, fitness, and thinness plans that don't work. But at least they are trying; men seem to be too macho to even try. It certainly isn't that the guys know the directions don't work, but rather they are stubborn about asking for directions in the first place. Both genders are bad, so please don't get mad at me for using Sally. (Plus, when I was thinking about driving and California, the song, "Mustang Sally" popped into my head.) It's just a story.

2. I am not an alarmist. The bad results of living the good life are real, though, and for those who want to make things better, I commend them.

3. The single biggest factor in our trio of excess weight, elevated cholesterol, and partially clogged arteries is the exorbitant amount of fat we have eaten throughout our lives. Depending on our age and just how bad things have been, we have taken in from 500,000 to as much as 1,000,000 grams of fat more than what our bodies have needed.

4. You can't run it off. For all practical purposes, a person who has eaten badly their whole life, who doesn't exercise, who is overweight with elevated cholesterol and partially clogged arteries, simply is not capable of exercising enough to burn off all the calories. Cannot do it. (Again, details to follow, so bear with me). But this is not as bad as it might seem, because there are solutions.

5. Chronically overweight people often eat less food than thin people. They do so as a result of decades of bad eating and dieting, not because of genes, heredity, or a slow metabolism.

These things are mentioned here to help support that while this book revolves around exercise and proper eating, these two areas have been so misrepresented that far too many people believe the wrong things. It is this book's premise that if we look at what correct eating means, and eat accordingly, and learn what exercise really is, and exercise, we can begin to reverse the negative effects of the good life. We have the right map.

What did I say?

I talk too much. It's better, then, that you read this book rather than talk to me about it, because reading will take less time and be easier to digest. Either way, I do not claim to be giving nutritional advice. I am not qualified to do that, so no where will you read me or hear me get into things such as the amounts and percentages of certain types of foods that a person should eat. Like X quantity of protein. Or anything else that pertains to specific nutritional information that only a credentialed person might put forth. So I'm disclaiming. All I am trying to do is to help people by giving some direction. When you see me write, for example, "eat lots of fruits and vegetables," I don't consider that nutritional advice. It is not worthy of that. It is not a revelation to anyone as far as I am concerned. Is that news to you, and is it something only a nutritionist is able to tell you? No and no. But I do write about how much fat people eat and should eat. But all that comes from the common place: the information that surrounds us.

This book is mostly about things you already know. I am only trying to encourage you to grow with the knowledge by understanding it better, with a bit of my own stuff thrown in.

Now You

This book only pertains to you. Don't look around, then, at others. Just check out where you are by getting the information you need (cholesterol level, etc.) and read along. The book is for you, and I wish you well.

Expansion of the Disclaimer

This is more disclaiming. Read it please, or I will feel slighted. Now, here goes. Just a little earlier I said I won't be giving nutritional advice, and I won't. However, as I also said, you will see me write endlessly about the ills of eating excess fat. I absolutely do not consider that nutritional advice, because I have seen, heard, and read literally hundreds if not thousands of times that eating excess fat is a terrible thing. Since I have come across it that much without even trying, I assume everyone else has also. We can't avoid the scream. Bob Dylan sang, "You don't need a weather man to know which way the wind blows." Our bodies need less than 10% of their calories from fat, as a fact, not opinion. We have been getting 35% to as much as 45% of our calories from fat. Fat is bad. I don't mean to sound like a simpleton, but there is no riddle here that requires a person with a college degree in nutrition to unravel. Most nutritionists couldn't unravel it anyway, which is a disgrace. It seems that nutritionists are still being trained to believe that we can safely get up to 30% of our calories from fat. If this sounds mixed up, it is. We need less than ten and the formally trained are saying thirty, and we all know fat is bad. Note what Dr. Dean Ornish writes in his book, *Eat More, Weigh Less*: "It's the excessive amounts of fat and cholesterol in your diet—that is, more than 10 percent of calories as fat—that lead to excess weight, heart disease, and other illnesses…Your body needs only about 4 to 6 percent of calories as fat…" I have a stack of other books to support Ornish. But I have to disclaim. If you question the amount of fat you should eat and believe you should follow a nutritionist because he or she is formally trained in nutrition, then do that. I suggest you also check with your doctor. If in doubt about anything regarding your health, go to your doctor.

To try to make all this even clearer, let me say this: if I see two sides, I can take sides. In our case here, one side I see says a lot of fat is OK, and the other side says it's not. Yet we keep eating more fat and getting heavier and ever more unhealthy. The correlation approaches 100%, as far as I am concerned. And everyone, for all practical purposes, knows excess fat is bad. So I chose.

Even though I am not a nutritionist and don't claim to be giving nutritional advice, I rant and rave about excess fat. If you ask me, or even demand me, and you even put me under the influence of truth serum (if there really is such a thing) or put me under hypnosis, to tell you what the recommended amounts of protein and carbohydrates are that a person should eat, I couldn't. I don't know. This is what I believe…don't eat excess fat, eat lots of fruits, vegetables, and grains, do a few other things with your eating as detailed later in Chapter 4, and all will be well. I also believe that everyone else knows all this.

Exercise is the other issue. Every adult, no matter what condition they think they are in, absolutely must see a doctor before starting on an exercise program. This isn't meant to scare you, it is just reality. There is no reason not to. Make sure you tell your doctor why. You are there not for a glance-over, but rather because you want to do everything possible to become healthy, fit, and thin. Therefore you are going to start exercising. Your ability to do that needs to be reviewed in detail by a doctor. Heart, cardiovascular system, the works. The plan then, is this: start eating right, see your doctor, finish this book, and get moving.

2

Fat Begets Fat…and Hypertension, Diabetes, Cancer, Strokes, Heart Attacks, and On and On, and Worse

Fat is the enemy, the problem, and the cause. It is not a part of the issue, it is the issue. You can only be fat, for all practical purposes, if you eat too much fat. Eating way too much fat, as most Americans do, leads not only to weight gain and obesity, but can cause hypertension, diabetes, various cancers, strokes, heart attacks, and more. It can even lead to premature death. It is that bad, and that simple. In 1910, the typical American got 20% of their calories from fat and wasn't fat. By 1980, the number stood at 40%, and most people were overweight with clogged arteries and elevated cholesterol, and the related ill-health was showing up everywhere. As we have seen, 20% is more than what our bodies need, so 40% is dramatically and dangerously too much, as our declining health and continually escalating weight prove.

From an article in the Chicago Tribune (2-5-95) titled "Silent killer threatens up to 45% of U.S. adult:" "After struggling for millions of years to escape the threat of famine and to make survival easier, humans are learning a cruel lesson about the good life: It's killing us." The article continues: "Diabetes…now strikes Americans at the rate of one new case every 52 seconds and threatens to overwhelm developing nations as they switch to Westernized lifestyles that emphasize rich foods and leisure."

Here are some enlightening words from the book *Fitness Without Exercise* by Bryant A. Stamford, Ph.D. and Porter Shimer: "If you were given the job of concocting a food component hazardous to human health, you would be hard pressed to come up with something more insidious than saturated fat...Next to cigarette smoking, excess dietary fat bears the burden of being the single most preventable cause of death that we face." The book goes on to explain that the typical American eats twelve times as much fat as the body requires. Not a little too much, or fifty percent too much, or way too much, but twelve times too much.

This "twelve times too much" is probably a surprise and a shock to most people, due to the fact that we have been flooded with so much bad information, to the point that the good has been washed away. Just look at the nutrition label the U.S. government requires be placed on all packaged foods. The label says to limit the amount of calories we get from fat to 30%, but our bodies need only 4% to 6%. So the federal government is telling us that to be good boys and girls, we can eat at least five times the amount of fat we need while at the same time the government recognizes that eating excess fat is bad. Couple this with the fact that most people get more than 30% of their calories from fat, regardless of the label, and it becomes clear why things are as bad as they are and why they keep getting worse.

I was gentle here too, because my editor told me to lighten things up. I deleted many other harsh statistics, so please don't think I was being overly dramatic in the opening of this chapter. Trust me, the situation is not good.

Amazing

I think I use the word amazing too much. But it is amazing that so many people do not know about the evils of eating too much fat. So here are some tidbits to help those who don't yet know and to reinforce it for those who do know:

> There are roughly twice as many calories in a gram of fat than in a gram of protein or a gram of carbohydrate.

> A person can cook a meal of pasta with sauce, corn, asparagus, and sourdough bread, consume just 800 calories and only 5 grams of fat, and wind up with a nice meal high in nutritional value. Or, that person can eat a typical American style helping of pizza, consume 2,000 calories and 80 grams of fat, and get fat, clog their arteries, and raise their cholesterol through the roof. Since a person needs only 15 to 20 grams of fat per day, the problem of 80 grams from the pizza is huge. And how about:

1. One donut: 13 grams of fat.

2. One cheeseburger: 36 grams of fat.

3. One order of fries: 19 grams of fat.

4. One milkshake: 27 grams of fat.

5. The numbers 2, 3, and 4 above, the cheeseburger, fries, and shake, are usually eaten at the same meal, so at one sitting, 82 grams of fat. Astronomical.

6. One breakfast of bacon, eggs, hash browns, and toast with butter, as recommended as a way to lose weight by some people in today's days of nonsense: 85 grams of fat.

And so forth. I don't mean to sound foolish, but I wish some other problems were as easy to fix as this. Like my golf swing. I scheduled another lesson to work on that. But you don't have to work on much with the eating right thing. Just first stop eating fat and then review Chapter 4 on eating right.

Epilogue

You might be asking, "But what about the different kinds of fat, like saturated and unsaturated? I keep hearing that one is OK and one is not?"

Good question, and yes, there is a difference, a big one. But too much attention has been paid to this. Saturated fat is the main problem. Some of the other fats are actually good for the body, and, in fact, our bodies need some fat to function properly. Most saturated fat comes from animal products, and everyone that eats too much fat essentially gets all the excess from animal fat, from meat, cheese, milk, butter, mayonnaise, sour cream, pizza, etc. Eating properly means virtually eliminating saturated fat, and that is not nearly as difficult as it might seem. It does not mean becoming a vegetarian. As I write this, I can smell dinner cooking. A few hours ago, I put the following in the crock pot: boneless, skinless, chicken breasts, tomato sauce, and canned tomatoes. It smells great. It will be served on rice and accompanied by fresh corn, fresh string beans, and sourdough bread. It will be delicious, filling, and nutritious. It has animal product but virtually no fat of any kind. For dessert, fresh peaches. Easy.

"It doesn't apply to me," said the hugely overweight guy.

The idea that things "can't happen to me" is human nature. A tragedy in another family, an illness elsewhere, whatever. We all think we are immune. But with our health most adult Americans are already a statistic. They have the three things that can, and usually do, lead to serious problems:

> Elevated cholesterol

> Excess weight

> Partially clogged arteries

The National Center of Health Statistics estimates that of people 40 years old and above, 80% of men and 70% of women are above their ideal weight (Chicago Tribune 5-8-00), and I believe those percentages are even higher and show up even earlier. The problems are likely present in people in their 20's. The percentage of people with elevated cholesterol and partially clogged arteries is also dramatically high.

OK, OK

The body needs a little fat as mentioned above. So you will eat fat, but the fat you eat will be almost exclusively of the non-saturated types. Whatever saturated fat you eat will be in very small quantities compared to what has been going on. Like instead of a cheeseburger, fries, and shake with at least 82 grams of fat, way too much of which is saturated, you might make chicken tacos using skinless white meat. Or very, very lean beef. So even though you will not and cannot and must not eat zero fat, the amount you will now eat is minuscule compared to the past. You couldn't eat zero fat anyway, even if you wanted to. Once you stop most of the saturated fat, you will have the problem resolved. And most means something like over 90% of it.

No fat to me still means no fat, because there will be no more big, gigantic helpings of fat. Absolutely none. Gone. Done.

Why Now

We dealt with this issue of eating excess fat before we got to the chapter on eating right (Chapter 4), because this fat thing is so overwhelmingly important. So much to the point that it can't be just a part of the whole. It is a "whole" on its own. No more fat.

3

Eat Less & Less, Weigh More & More. In Other Words, Diets Don't Work

"It's easy to lose weight, I do it all the time," said the Fat Lady.

A Digression

I like digressions. They break things up and offer hope of more interesting things. Like in school when we were kids, any pause in the usual, boring flow always held out the possibility of excitement. Maybe, instead of studying math, we were going to see a film. Any topic would do. So, I will add digressions here and there, to help hold your interest.

Like the matter of eating excess fat needing to be attended to before we get to the larger area of eating right, so too the issue of dieting needs addressing. Without fully understanding the terrible effects of dieting, we cannot go on. So this chapter on dieting is also presented before the chapter on eating right (Chapter 4).

Back To It

When I was preparing to write this chapter on diets, a title jumped out at me. It seemed so obvious. Since most overweight people have been on diet after diet, for years and even decades, and all these people keep getting heavier and heavier, it seemed perfectly clear that diets don't work. So, the title to the chapter would have to be, "Diets Don't Work." But something in the back of my mind wasn't right. A bit more thought revealed the truth: diets do work, all of them. What I first thought was a no-brainer title for the chapter was completely wrong, because every diet ever undertaken works, in the short term, as a result of what a diet is:

> Diet: Short term food deprivation undertaken for the purpose of losing weight, after which the diet is ended and all the lost weight is regained plus more, so the dieter becomes heavier than before the diet started. (This definition isn't out of a dictionary. I wrote it based on reality.)

By definition then, diets work. The list of diets is effectively endless, with more being invented daily, and to name a fraction of the total would fill up dozens of pages. Ridiculous things that I won't insult your intelligence with, but haven't we all heard of The Grapefruit Diet? I do believe that if you just eat grapefruit you will lose weight. You might die, but the point is, the diet works. If grapefruit, why not bananas, apples, string beans, potatoes, or whatever? Nonsense.

There are countless diets, because, as the definition of a diet points out, all diets fail in the long run, so overweight people continually need a different diet. There is always someone standing by with the next useless one, and there will be no end to this until people learn that the correct way to good health and correct weight is not through dieting. Without knowing this people are doomed to continued problems.

It would seem that this diet/get heavier cycle would have been recognized long ago, but people haven't seen it. Here is perhaps why:

> 1. The fact that diets work in the short term makes people believe that the weight gain seen after the diet ends is the result of personal weakness. Diet promoters know this and capitalize on it by marketing the next new, miracle diet by saying things such as, "This time you won't fail." So people try the next diet with the same result, over and over, failing each time, thinking it is their fault.

2. People diet, because it seems to make sense that severely restricting the amount of food eaten will lead to weight loss. (We will see soon that just the opposite is the case…which is the point of this chapter.)

3. People are always being told of someone who lost a lot of weight on such and such a diet and that it was easy.

4. We are literally inundated with diet plans. Everywhere we look we see a new one. They all work, too, for a few minutes anyway, and most of the advertisements are very convincing.

So, let's put all this together and see what has caused the problems.

Why, Why, Why Diets Cause Weight Gain Over Time

The human body is magnificent. It wants to be healthy, and it tries hard to protect itself from disease and illness. It wants to function properly all the time, and it wants to stay in a healthy, normal state. It fights off change. When you start doing things to your body that are significant departures from what you normally do, the body will resist the changes, which leads us to the "why?"

Here is what happens, in non-technical terms. A person is overweight, has been for years (and often for decades) as a result of eating horribly, which means skipping meals, and when eating, wolfing down huge quantities of high-fat foods. Since bad eating turns into the norm, the body becomes overweight and accepts being overweight. It gets used to it. Then along comes a diet, and all of a sudden, without warning, a dramatic change occurs. The body fights it off, but the dieter continues. The body starts to worry, because compared to what it has been used to, it is starving. It is literally afraid for its life, because, as we know, people have actually died from diets. In defense, the body, when it gets this drastically reduced quantity of food, uses just enough of it to keep functioning and stores the rest as fat for what looks like an emergency. The body becomes very efficient at this, so when the dieter quits the diet (remember the definition of a diet where it says that all diets come to an end) the body needs fewer calories then it did before the diet began. As the intake of calories now increases above what was eaten during the diet, the body continues to use as few calories as possible and stores the rest as fat, and therefore, now an even higher proportion of calories eaten are stored as fat. The body begins to gain back the weight that was lost during the diet, and when all that lost weight is regained, extra weight even beyond that is added, because of this new need for less. The body then winds up heavier than before the diet started. This action is repeated regularly over the years, resulting in an ever heavier, ever more unhealthy person.

That is it, but to help those people who are reluctant to accept such a non-technical analysis from me, here is a more scientific one from two dietitians who obviously understand things: "Low-calorie diets double the enzymes that make and store fat as a form of biological compensation to help the body store more energy, or fat, after dieting." (From the book *Intuitive Eating, A Recovery Book for the Chronic Dieter* by registered dietitians Evelyn Tubole and Elyse Resch, as quoted by the Chicago Tribune, May 8, 1996.)

I want to make things as clear as I am able to, and this information as to why dieting causes weight gain over time hopefully accomplishes that objective. It was short, to the point, and from two directions. Since dieting causes weight gain over time, don't diet.

If you go on a diet, no matter what you do during that diet, you will gain back all the weight you lose, plus you will gain even more weight beyond that. Guaranteed.

"The Government Did What? You've Got To Be Kidding!"

Since we know that dieting causes weight gain over time, we should see to it that this information is made available to everyone. The U.S. government, however, is doing just the opposite. In the May 31, 2000 Chicago Tribune, there is a picture of two overweight government workers, Health Secretary Donna Shalala and Agriculture Secretary Dan Glickman, alongside the headline of an article titled "U.S. to test 2 rival diets in fight against obesity." Here we now have the U.S. government promoting the idea that diets might cure obesity, when in fact we already know just the opposite, that dieting contributes to, and even causes, weight gain and obesity. The article says, "Worried that Americans are doing the wrong thing to lose weight, the government has decided to test two of the nation's most popular diets…to see which is the more effective and safer way to drop the pounds." Stupid, yes, because the biggest of the "wrong" things people are doing to lose weight is to diet.

Our problems are guaranteed to keep getting worse unless we stop the bad eating, the dieting, and the nonsense such as we get from the government. Eat right and exercise, if you want to become healthy, fit, and thin. Do not go on a diet, because:

Diets Cause Weight Gain Over Time

This knowledge about how dieting actually causes weight gain over time is some of the best news we could possibly have. We can't fail anymore, because we won't be doing something that guarantees failure.

4

Masticating Correctly…and Ole' Olestra

Bacon and eggs for breakfast with a donut for a mid-morning snack, and for lunch two cheeseburgers, a large order of fries, and a shake. A candy bar in the afternoon, then for dinner a steak with a baked potato loaded with butter and sour cream, lots of bread and butter, followed by a large piece of rich, fat-filled pie with fat-filled ice cream on top. Eat like this every day, and you will become healthy, fit, and thin. Oops, I mean fat, then dead. I get mixed up with all the asinine information some people are throwing at us these days.

The Real Story

There seems to be no end to what people will believe if the information promises an easy path to good health and thinness. In fact, as ludicrous as it should be, there are people who believe eating properly means eating about like what was described above in the opening paragraph. For real. Yet the real story goes like this: "…American eating habits…are a disaster. They are so far afield from what we were evolved to eat that most of the diseases we see are linked to what people eat and other aspects of their life-style." (From the book, *The 10% Solution for A Healthy Life*, by Raymond Kurzweil.)

It is so bad, that if it wasn't a reality, it would be hard even to imagine anything so awful. Yet people ignore sound advice and embrace the ridiculous. It is just about impossible for me to have a casual conversation with people about nutrition, because people have such bad information and believe so strongly in it. But the truth is, our eating habits have eroded dramatically, and for all practical purposes we are doing nothing about them. We might think we are, but we are not. We need to fix things, and we can, because it is not difficult. But first we need to face reality.

Reality

We will see throughout this book the damages our lifestyle has created and how people relish the ludicrous in terms of remedies. But there is more. People actually fool themselves even further. Skipping meals, which is bad, is one way. Also, most adults declare they are eating better than they used to, and they base their position on small, meaningless changes such as eating low-fat cookies instead of traditional high-fat ones, and eating and drinking other lighter versions of food and drink. These changes add up to so little that the effect is nil, and the damage keeps getting worse. The reality, then, looks like this:

1. We are eating more in terms of calories than we used to, about 200 more per day than in 1970.

2. We "look" at the labels on the food we buy, but we still buy way too many things that are bad.

3. We still eat way, way too much fat.

What To Do

Piece of cake. Really. (Chocolate with white frosting is my first choice.) We are just going to eat right. However, while most people pretty much know what that means, we have gotten so far away from it that when we do make small moves back towards eating right, we think we are all the way back. But we are not even close. We can see this if we think about eating properly on a scale from 1 to 10, with the worst at 1 and 10 the best. If we are at 2 or 3 and we do a few things better for a day or two, we believe we have moved up the scale to 7 or 8, and we think we are eating right. Switching from large fries to medium fries with our cheeseburgers would be an example, but doing so is absolutely no improvement. The bottom line is that we eat about as badly as possible, we are at the low end of the scale, and we need to get to the other end, quickly.

Sudden, Dramatic, and Complete

There is just one way to go about changing from bad eating to proper eating, and that is to do it all at once. No little steps as many suggest. I am convinced it has to be sudden, dramatic, and complete, because the little changes people have made have just not added up to anything meaningful. For example, most people have gotten around 40% of their calories from fat. Some of these people, in an attempt at eating better, have cut that down to 30% or so for some short period of time. Since even 30% is still way too much, nothing improved. It has to be all or nothing. Let's see what the "all" means.

There is a common set of guidelines for proper eating that shows up most everywhere, and it goes about like this:

> Eat lots of fruits, vegetables, and whole grains.

> Drink lots of water.

> Eat at least three meals a day.

> Limit the amount of calories you get from fat to 30% of total calories.

> Limit the amount of refined sugar.

This set of recommendations pretty much summarizes most of what we have heard for a long time, and for the most part it is all good information except for the very bad bit about the fat. The fat thing is so bad it negates most everything else. But the guidelines, otherwise, are about right, sound bland, are usually not detailed enough, and are pretty much ignored by everyone. Since they are close in accuracy, though, I can only go basically along the same route. I don't want to lose anyone because of the blandness, though, so I am going to attempt to expand and add to make for interest, clarification, and do-ability. I will also be brief, and at the end of each item I will add a "Twist," to help make it clear. Please, even if the twist is not much of a twist, take it seriously. But first:

The Don'ts

When you see my agenda that outlines how to eat, a lot of it will be familiar. However, since we have been unable or unwilling to pattern our eating habits accordingly, I want to smooth things out and try to make them easier to deal with. In this regard, let me first list the major things a person trying to make things better absolutely should not eat. You probably know this list, or most of it anyway, but I want you to focus on it so you can get serious with it. That should make it easier to concentrate on the do's.

The first don't is don't get mad at me for reciting the obvious. I am only trying to help and to get a mindset going. Now, let's look at the following list of foods that should not be eaten, at all, until you become healthy, fit, and thin. Once that happens you might have some of these things from time to time, because some here and there will do no harm. Without completely cutting all this stuff out for now, though, progress will be virtually impossible:

> Pizza (it is full of fat and extremely high in calories).

> Beef (extra lean in small quantities if you must).

> Donuts, cakes, pies, and all such stuff that is full of fat.

> Ice cream that is full of fat.

> French fries.

> All other fried foods.

> Fast food (Just about all of it is high fat. There are exceptions, so just be careful.).

> Bacon and eggs and all other high-fat products that come from things that walk.

> Eat nothing high in fat.

> Anything else you might think is bad, because if you think it is bad, it probably is bad.

That is the bulk of it, and it is easy to see that it is all about fat. Now let's look at the do's, the directions on how to go about this eating right thing. Some of the do's start with the word don't, but you'll know what I mean.

1. Stop Eating Fat

Sorry, but I feel a need to be relentless. Whenever I begin to talk about eating right, the first thing I say is, "Stop eating fat." The excess fat we have been eating for decades is what has caused most of our health and weight problems.

The idea of just cutting back on fat as suggested by so many "authorities" (read: the U.S. government and far too many of the credentialed), rather than stopping altogether, will not work, because we eat so much of it, but need so little.

This "Stop Eating Fat" was listed in the "Don't," because it is a don't. It is listed again here because of its importance.

Twist #1: Stop means stop.

2. Eat Somewhere Around Zero Simple Carbohydrates

Simple carbohydrates are things such as table sugar, complex carbohydrates are in whole foods such as fruits, vegetables, and whole grains. (Simple is a starch refined, and complex is a starch in its natural, unrefined state.) Whatever forms the simple stuff comes in, regular, reduced, or low, the cookies, cakes, pies, donuts, candy, soft drinks and so on have to stop. If you think it is junk, it probably is junk.

Twist #2: The twist here is the completeness. Stop all the simple carbs. Anything and everything.

3. Eat Fruits, Veggies, and Grains

Boring. Not a chance. Learn how to serve them and enjoy them. I am not a cook, so there are no recipes here, but there are many books to show you how.

I think most people understand what this fruit, grain, and vegetable thing is all about, but they don't do it, or they don't do it nearly enough. I have seen people at their jobs who bring in a banana that sometimes gets eaten and sometimes doesn't. The bananas are brought in because people know they should eat more fruit, but seldom do the banana-bringers do it often enough to do any good, and most of these people are doing many other things wrong, to the point where the occasional banana does nothing. These people most assuredly skipped breakfast, thereby setting up the body for fat storage later when they do eat, making the effort to bring the banana a waste. So, eat a lot of fruit, all day, every day, just as we've been advised to do for as long as we can remember.

As far as veggies go, there are endless ways to take advantage of the healthy benefits, besides just eating them raw as snacks. Get a crock pot (a slow cooker), some recipes, and toss in a load of vegetables.

Many nights I make a combination vegetable and fruit juice, with my favorite being made with carrots, celery, apples, parsley, and garlic. The taste is phenomenal, the nutritional value sky high, and sometimes that juice, along with a bowl of rice, is dinner.

Each morning, as only a part of my breakfast, I make a fruit shake: two bananas, an apple, and an orange in the blender with at least one other carbohydrate, like other fruit or jam, with milk. That's five servings of fruit to start the day, with another two to five servings throughout the day. Veggies at every dinner and some as snacks in the afternoon and usually some at lunch. Whole grain cereals and breads.

Twist #3: Eat more fruits and vegetables than you have ever seen recommended.

<u>4. Don't Skip Meals</u>

Our bodies are the most magnificent and fascinating things in the world, and we should take care of them. Our mental and physical well-beings are at stake. Since our bodies are so complex and capable of so much, it follows that they require specific, on-going, regular maintenance. Like the right foods, in the right quantities, at the right times, meaning in part that we can't skip meals. But most people do.

The meal that is skipped most frequently, by far, is breakfast, and of all the excuses for doing so, a lack of time, trying to lose weight, and not being hungry in the morning dominate the list. But none of these excuses are valid, because breakfast is just too important.

We have heard all of our lives that breakfast is the most important meal of the day, and it is, but we still skip it. Since our body must have an ongoing supply of nutrition, and by the time breakfast time rolls around we haven't eaten for ten to twelve hours, food becomes critical. Not eating breakfast affects us negatively in both the short term and long term. The importance of eating breakfast is so overwhelming that if you want to become healthy, fit and thin, breakfast is a must.

Breakfast, of course, should be all good stuff, like fruit and cereal with fiber and without the sugar coatings. Throw in some protein, even peanut butter, on toast or on saltines. Eat a lot. For those of you who say, "I'm not hungry in the morning," your lack of hunger comes from the fact that your body has gotten used to no breakfast. When you were a kid you were starving in the morning. The body adapts and you have taught it not to be hungry in the morning.

That thing about not having time in the morning to eat just doesn't hold water. You can do anything you want, for all practical purposes, and I am not being trite. The "for all practical purposes" means that you will not likely be able to take up basketball and become a better basketball player than Michael Jordan, or take up golf and become a better golfer than Tiger, but finding time for breakfast doesn't rank near such achievements. I know a couple who "didn't have time" for things, like for eating right and exercising, so they stopped watching TV and picked up over a dozen hours every week. They started getting more done, going to bed earlier, and getting up earlier to both exercise and eat breakfast. No time is just no excuse. Most people spend around 1,000 hours every year staring at that vast area of meaningless, nothingness known as television. Turn it off.

Juice and coffee is not breakfast. Nor is just toast and juice. Eat, and enjoy. You will be doing yourself a huge favor.

> Twist #4: Skip no meals. None. The better you eat the harder it will become to miss a meal. I can't skip a meal, because I get too hungry, even in the morning. Especially in the morning. I'm starving in the morning.

5. Don't Eat Too Much

The proclamation, "Don't eat too much," might seem obvious, but the message is in the details. The first one is that, on average, we eat about 200 calories per day more than we did thirty years ago. This math, when totaled up, might surprise you, because if a person was to be eating properly and as a result was ideal in weight and then began eating 200 calories more than that per day for thirty years, that person would gain 625 pounds. Of course no one has really gained that many pounds, because a lot of other factors come into play, but the basic theme is scary and the message clear: we eat too much, way too much.

Those 200 more calories per day equate to 73,000 more calories per year and 2,190,000 more over that thirty year period. The mystery is solved. Just eat right, and do so by adhering to the following:

> Eat no fat.

> Eat a large breakfast with all kinds of good stuff, like cereal, fruit, and protein.

> Eat a healthy lunch, without stuffing yourself.

> Eat as little for dinner as you can get by with.

> Eat all good food, with emphasis on more food early in the day rather than later.

> Eliminate junk.

Twist #5: The twist here is that this isn't about portion control. It's about eating right. The portions will then take care of themselves.

6. Eat Fish

Another great idea we have heard about forever, but don't often do. Fish is good for us and low in fat. There are a lot of different fish to choose from and many ways to prepare it. So instead of high-fat meat, try some low-fat fish recipes, and you will benefit greatly. Not once in a while either, but frequently, from now on.

Twist #6: Once in a while, or even once a week, won't do. Everyone needs to have fish two to three times a week, or more. Be sure to use only low-fat recipes. There is no reason to eat healthy fish prepared in fat.

7. Slow Down

We eat too fast which often causes us to eat too much. Did you know that it takes twenty minutes for your brain to register fullness? Do you ever go to a restaurant for dinner and soon after arriving you begin to eat bread or rolls and a salad, and then thirty minutes after you sat down and you are done with the bread and salad and you are waiting for your main course to arrive, you say, "I'm full?" Such an occasion, that of being forced to slow down, illustrates that if we give our brain a chance to catch up with our mouth, we will eat less.

Twist #7: How many times have you gone to eat a snack before a meal and were told, "Don't ruin your appetite." Well, ruin it, with something healthy.

8. Don't Eat Salad

Not really, but we have to do it right. If we do it wrong like the following anecdote shows, we should leave the salad alone.

One day I was at a soup and sandwich place for lunch and near the ordering counter was a refrigerated display of salads and dressings. One foil packet caught my attention, because it said, "Light Ranch Salad Dressing." It was called light, because instead of having 140 calories like their normal ranch dressing, it had 110. It also had 14 grams of fat, which is not far from what a person needs for an entire day, and wasted on a silly little packet of salad dressing. (The 110 calories is way too much, also.) Guess who it is that eats such stuff, by the way? Overweight people trying to lose weight. Crazy.

Overweight people usually don't eat breakfast, then they might have a bad snack like a donut mid-morning if hunger and opportunity come together, then some of them eat a salad with dressing like that just mentioned for lunch. Or they eat a salad loaded with high fat food such as hard-boiled eggs, cheese, and meat. All terrible ways to go about things, since most overweight people are eating salad because of their excess weight.

Salads should be eaten regularly, because they are very nutritional when properly prepared. In our house we eat them more and more often, and we keep getting more creative in their preparation. As for what we top them off with, there are numerous no fat and low fat dressings that taste excellent and that are low in calories.

Twist #8: Eat salads all the time, but do it right.

<u>9. Don't Drink Things With Calories</u>

What a waste of calories. Not that calories matter, as we will see in Chapter 5, but far too many of our calories come from things we drink. Water is good for us, it has no calories, and we don't drink anywhere near enough of it. Compare water with the following:

> 12 ounces of apple juice, 180 calories

> 12 ounces of peach nectar, 200 calories

> 12 ounces of grape juice, 240 calories

Since most people don't come close to drinking the proper amount of water, the plan needs to be to load up on water while cutting back to near zero on drinks with calories. Save the calories for good, nutritious food.

Twist #9: Drink, drink, and then drink, water. (A note about this water thing. Drinking a lot of water will not cause a person to lose weight, nor will it reduce a person's appetite. But too many people believe such things. We have all probably seen overweight people at work start having extra water on hand, and this comes from the losing-weight misconception. Drink a lot of water, because water is critical to good health. That is reason enough, and the only reason.)

Shoot The Messengers

We have to stop paying attention to all the bad information that routinely bombards us. We won't really shoot anyone (another official disclaimer), but the point is well made, I do believe. Instead, we will ignore, and the ignoring will focus on things such as the following:

Messenger #1: The U.S. Government.

A very bad thing happened to our health when the U.S. government mandated that all foods require the nutritional content label that we are all now familiar with. The problem is that the label says we can get up to 30% of our calories from fat. As we see throughout this book, fat is the enemy, and 30% is way too much. It turns out that the government's cure is actually the cause. Shame on them.

Messenger #2: The Food Companies.

Stop listening to them and you will stop being persuaded by them. Too much of what they have to say is terrible, as a few examples will show:

> Some time ago, Burger King started offering a breakfast sandwich called the Breakfast Buddy®. I'm not sure they sell it any more, but it's irrelevant whether they do or not. One of those little buddies contained 16 grams of fat. You know the old saying, "With friends like that, who needs enemies." Eat enough of those and your buddy might cause you some real trouble. Please note that I am not picking on Burger King. The fact is this: Burger King, McDonald's, Dunkin' Donuts, the pizza places, and all the rest are only offering what people want, and doing a great job. People want to eat fat, so fat is available in abundance, everywhere. We asked for what we got. Fat and junk. Breakfast Buddies and all their pals.

> I have in front of me a newspaper ad for Maruchan® Ramen. It has a "babe" holding a bowl of the noodles, implying that hot "chicks" eat that stuff. Or I guess that if you are female and not hot, you will become hot by eating this product. The ad says, "Get in shape for spring with easy to prepare Maruchan Ramen…" Ridiculous. Each package makes two servings, and each serving contains 8 grams of fat. I believe

most people, even sexy women, when they eat this food eat a whole package, which means this purported good stuff supplies 16 grams of fat in just one bowl. Way too much.

There are endless other examples. If the food has excess fat in it, don't eat it, regardless of what the food company says.

Messenger #3: Weight-loss Plans, Scams and Schemes

As seen elsewhere in this book, as well as in that part of our heads that deals with reality, diets are bad because they actually cause weight gain over time. The promoters of diets are notorious for hype and false promises. Ignore them, too.

…and Ole' Olestra®

If this wasn't real, I wouldn't believe it. It comes right out of the "Are we nuts?" file. Olestra is a fat substitute that was developed to add to food, such as chips, so the food can be sold as low fat, reduced-fat, or fat-free. Frito-Lay became the first company to use Olestra when it began selling low fat and no fat versions of its Lay's ®, Ruffles ®, Doritos ® and Tostitos ® chips. This synthetic chemical (brand name Olean ®) is derived from sugar and vegetable oil. It tastes and cooks like fat but passes through the body undigested because its molecules are so large. While this sounds good up to this point, there is a catch. It seems that, as compared to chips made the regular way, the ones with Olestra can cause people to develop gastrointestinal problems. Things like cramps and diarrhea. It is so bad that the following information label has to appear on foods that contain the product

"Olestra may cause abdominal cramping and loose stools."

But surprise. People are buying the stuff and eating it anyway, and they are doing so in spite of revelations such as:

>…the following quote from Michael Jacobson, the director of the Center for Science in the Public Interest, a group

known for watching out for unhealthy foods: "Here's something being added to the food supply by multi-billion dollar corporations that's making people poop in their pajamas. It's insane!" (U.S. News & World Report, May 5, 1997)

>...a 37 year old male who ate a small bowl of chips made with Olean spent all night in his bathroom and was sick for two more days. "It was like food poisoning but much more severe" he said (Chicago Tribune, July 2, 1996).

>...Michael Jacobson again, at the Indiana Press Club, showed a fake dog food can with the loose-stools-and-cramping olestra label while he asked the question, "If you saw that, would you give it to your dog?" The amazing thing about this is that I doubt there is one person who would buy such a product for their dog, but guess what...shortly after release in a test market in central Indiana the chips called WOW! ® became the largest selling chips in the area" (U.S. News & World Report, May 5, 1997).

Eating right really can be easy, and a big part of the "easy" is staying away from the ridiculous.

The Dilemma

We have a dilemma. Or more accurately, some might think we do. If a person looks at the guidelines I have outlined and sees that eating right means eating three wholesome meals a day and not skipping meals and eating lots of fruits, vegetables, grains, and fish, etc., it might look like more food will be eaten than what that person has been eating. So weight will be gained. Some sorting out, then, is called for.

Most people have been eating so poorly for so long that confusion should exist. Skipping meals, particularly not eating breakfast then having something small like a salad for lunch, then eating a large dinner regardless of whether it is high fat, high calorie or something healthy, usually leads people to think they are not eating a lot. Yet as shown elsewhere in this book, such eating often causes weight gain, even if the total calories might be less over time than that of a thin person who eats correctly. However, if an overweight person begins to eat correctly, which means eating the right foods, eaten at the right times in the right quantities, and an exercise program is implemented, that person will begin the process of becoming healthy, fit, and thin. There is no dilemma, because the answer is always the same, eat right and exercise. Calories might not matter anyway, as we will see in the next chapter.

No More Fine Dining!

That would probably ruin the lives of my wife and myself and do serious damage to the economy here in Chicago. Seriously though, eating out at restaurants way above the fast food fare is a problem. So let's talk about it.

Eating fine food is one of the great pleasures of life. Care has to be taken, though, because as far as I am concerned, the amount of calories and quantity of fat are often so high as to be incalculable. Therefore, you will have to eliminate such dining until you are well along the path to better things. If you must, due to some type of social or business reason, try real hard to do good. You know the deal. As little fat as possible.

Another Song

Remember the song, "Do you know the way to San Jose?" How about to Seattle, as in Seattle Sutton's Healthy Eating®. Seattle Sutton, R.N., B.S.N., is a registered nurse, turned entrepreneur. Her company sells food. All you need, all meals, just about.

The remarkable aspects about the program are the total of what it does and the simplicity through which it does it. Just by taking a couple minutes to place a weekly order, you get 21 fully-prepared meals that are:

- calorie controlled

- low in fat and cholesterol

- sodium restricted

- nutritionally balanced

- tasty

Yes, calorie controlled. (There are two calorie levels to choose from, 1,200 and 2,000.) I write a lot about calories not being important, and when I do so, I am just trying to make a point. Our eating habits are so bad that the amount of calories has not been important. If you skip breakfast, have a donut for a mid-morning snack, then nothing the rest of the day until dinner when you have fat junk, you will become overweight, your arteries will start to get clogged up, and your cholesterol will become elevated, even if you eat in total no more than the "recommended" amount of calories. The bottom line is that eating right means the right foods, in the right quantities, at the right times, on a consistent basis. So once you start eating right, of course calories count. Now, with Seattle Sutton's Healthy Eating, there is an easy way to do everything right.

I can confirm the tasty part, because I tried Seattle Sutton's Healthy Eating as part of my research for this book. I had come to realize how difficult it is for many people to eat right. Even with the best of intentions, doing so seems to be virtually impossible. The time to plan, shop, and prepare meals evidently doesn't exist for many. Since my bottom line is helping people, I went looking for ways to do that and found one. The best one possible. I tried the program, and I learned that everything Seattle Sutton says is true, and more. The "and more" part is amazing. This program might well go down as one of the best things since sliced bread, and the bread is included.

If you are lucky enough to have access to Seattle Sutton's Healthy Eating, try it. Ms. Sutton started in the Chicago area, and her company has grown to include parts of Nebraska, Wisconsin, Iowa, Indiana, and Minnesota. The company keeps growing, as you would expect with something this good, valuable, and unique, so if it is not in your area yet, cross your fingers; maybe it will be down the road.

5

Calories Don't Count. No, Calories Do Count. Wait. What I Really Want To Say Is: Yes, Overweight People Often Eat Less Than Thin People

Here is how it first hit me that many overweight people eat less than thin people. I found myself talking to a young woman who was around twenty-five years old, and she was extremely overweight. It came up in our conversation that I was writing this book, and she became both interested and distressed, because her mother had been giving her a hard time about her weight. The young woman told me that just a few days prior to our talk, the mother, during dinner, saw the daughter eat something and said, "You know that has too much fat in it, and you shouldn't eat it. I would never eat that!" The daughter was embarrassed and felt bad. She didn't want to be overweight, but since no matter what she did to try to lose weight, she kept getting heavier, discouragement and guilt ruled her every waking hour, and she was just plain miserable. The real issue here, though, is that the mom is even heavier than the daughter, and had been for as long as the daughter could remember. Mom had been obese for going on thirty years, her entire adult life, yet she thought she knew enough to advise her daughter regarding what to eat and what not to eat. Amazing.

The mom might very well know a lot about calories and the fat content in food, like many overweight people. I have often said that there are overweight people who know how many calories are in the chair they are sitting on. But that chair information has about as much value as knowing how much fat the donut had that was eaten mid-morning by this same overweight person as a substitute for breakfast. As is written in Chapter 4 about eating properly, most overweight people eat in such a way that they are guaranteed to keep getting heavier. These people diet, skip meals, and do other abnormal things in an effort to lose weight. While some of what they do might make sense in isolation, in the end they make matters worse. For example, it would seem that skipping meals, and therefore eliminating all calories for certain periods of time, would cause weight loss. However, skipping a meal causes the body to think you are starving it, so it gets very efficient with the calories it does finally get. Since the meals most frequently missed are breakfast and lunch, by dinner time the body has gone 24 hours with little or no food, so it uses just enough calories from dinner to sustain itself, and stores the rest as fat. The body gets used to this routine and becomes ever more efficient at adjusting to the skipped meals while becoming a great storer of fat, and wham, constant weight gain over time while eating fewer calories over time. In other words, overweight people often eat less than thin people; therefore, calories are not the issue. It is that basic.

On the other end of the skipping-meal phenomenon are the people who eat zillions of calories. They eat tons of food that is loaded with fat and high in calories at almost every meal, every day. These people are obviously overweight and unhealthy. So, at both ends of the calorie scale, people have the same problems. Forget calories. If you want to be healthy, fit, and thin, eat right and exercise, and please learn to ignore overweight people with nutritional advice.

Or, Maybe Calories Do Count

It just seems that calories should count, wouldn't you say? It is hard to imagine that calories are not important, because it appears to make so much sense. The literature overwhelmingly supports the validity of the calories-in vs. calories-out formula, and most books and programs revolve around that common recipe. And, of course, most of the "credentialed" believe so. But it doesn't hold, for all practical purposes. Here is further evidence that it doesn't. As we saw earlier, the average American today eats 200 more calories than what the average American ate in 1970. If calories-in/calories-out worked, such a person would weigh 625 pounds more than they did in 1970, and obviously this is not even near the case. Americans today certainly weigh more than they did back then, but not by over a quarter ton! This not-gaining-625-pounds thing certainly cannot be said to be offset by exercise, because the average American moves less today than in 1970. Besides, if the calories-in/calories-out thing worked, and the weight was not gained because the average American actually did exercise it off, doing so would have required the equivalent of running nearly 22,000 miles, and most everyone would have had to have done that. How many people do you know have run 22,000 miles? (Besides Forrest Gump.)

Calories Clarification

Every where we look, we see proof that negates the calories-in vs. calories-out formula. While the formula should work (we think), it is obvious it doesn't when reality is investigated. So how can I be right and most everyone else wrong? Go back to perspective. If a person eats right and has done so for a significant amount of time and is therefore healthy and of a normal weight, I would expect that the formula would work. But the people this book is geared towards, people who have never exercised and who have not been eating correctly for a very long time, will not properly respond to changes in calories and/or movement until they begin an on-going, regular program of eating right and exercising. And this will work only if such changes are sudden, dramatic, complete, and for some length of time, enough time to get the body reacting in a normal, positive manner.

So please don't let the calorie thing drive what you do. Eating right by definition will limit calories, and exercise will take care of the rest.

"How Many?"

I really don't want to talk about how many calories a person should eat, because we need to eat as if calories don't count. I don't count calories, and I never have. And I don't want you counting calories. Plus, I don't know how many calories a person should eat anyway. Because I don't need to know. Nor do you. Just eat right and exercise. Doing so will help make life good, the day great, and the head strong. Remember, calories don't count, but good eating habits do.

6

Metabolism: The Slow & The Fast, and It Doesn't Matter

What a nice word, metabolism. It sounds strong, and we all have one. But does it matter? I believe most people think it does, but it doesn't. Furthermore, this is also good news, because it is one more thing we can ignore as we get on with becoming healthy, fit, and thin.

Metabolism is usually thought of in its basic form of a person having either a slow one or a fast one, but the word actually refers to many complex activities that take place within the body. Since I am not interested in even the simple form, I won't even touch the complicated. The simple, though, has to be dealt with just to discard it, because it can get in the way.

In the simplest form, metabolism refers to the rate at which the body uses energy (burns calories), so that one person may naturally use more energy (burn more calories) than another person doing the same activity, whether that be just sitting, running, or whatever. Overweight people use the terms slow and fast metabolism to suit their needs by rationalizing how such and such a thin person is thin just because they are lucky enough to have a fast metabolism, while the overweight person talking is heavy purely because he or she had the bad luck to have been born with a slow metabolism. It is unfortunate that so many overweight people believe this, because doing so gives them an excuse for being overweight and not even attempting to solve their problem. To help such people, we need to take a look and see exactly why this whole metabolism thing is meaningless. Then we will look at the one exception that pertains to everyone. This exception is very important, but happily easy to deal with.

The Meaningless Part

Meaningless, because if a person eats right and exercises, he or she will be healthy, fit, and thin. The degree to which one person's metabolism might vary from the norm will not be enough to offset those two good things. Here's why. The body needs a certain amount of calories to function, so one cannot become overweight unless that person consumes more calories than they burn. (This does not conflict with what was written in the previous chapter about the calories-in/calories-out formula not being valid, because there we were talking about it not applying to people who have been eating incorrectly and not exercising for significant periods of time.) If their metabolism is slow, the amount of calories needed is lower, and if that amount of calories is not exceeded and is obtained from proper food eaten in a correct manner, body weight will not and cannot be elevated. If the metabolism is high, and as a result more calories are consumed, but not in excess of what the body needs, and those calories are the right ones eaten at the right times in the right quantities, no excess weight can occur. To help clarify, let's look at both cases:

1. If person "A" starts off at a normal weight and has a body that requires 1600 calories per day to supply all necessary energy, and that person eats properly and consumes 1600 calories per day, weight will remain constant. The body cannot make something out of nothing, so if the correct 1600 calories goes in the correct way and 1600 calories gets used, no change can take place. No weight can be gained.

2. If person "B," who also starts off at a normal weight, has a higher metabolism than person "A," so that "B" needs 2000 calo-

ries per day, and if "B" consumes no more than 2000 calories per day, again by eating properly, no weight gain will ensue.

It really is this simple. Therefore, a person's rate of metabolism is irrelevant. If you want to be healthy, fit, and thin, you eat right as explained in the chapter on eating, and a part of eating right means eating no more than what your body needs based on your metabolism and movement, regardless of whether one or both are slow, fast, or whatever. That is why, if you have your eyes on a couple cookies, and if eating those cookies will cause you to gain weight because the calories in them will put you over what your body needs, don't eat the cookies.

I hope you see the good news in all this, because it means that if you are overweight and you do what is necessary to lose the excess weight, you can keep it off by not eating any more than what your body needs. Or more to the point, by eating correctly as is repeated throughout this book. I have to make this distinction, because in the final analysis, the primary issue is not calories but eating properly. So, in order to avoid confusion, the point about metabolism as it pertains to overweight people who contribute their excess weight to a naturally slow metabolism is this: maintaining an ideal weight, after that ideal weight is achieved by proper eating and exercise, can be kept constant if a person then continues to eat correctly and does not exceed the amount of calories the body needs. Correct eating means correct foods at the right times in the proper amounts. And it means no fat. This could mean that a person who has been overweight for a long time, who has eaten improperly and gone on diet after diet and skipped meals, and who has in total done everything wrong for decades, might, after eating correctly and exercising for a long enough period to lose all the excess weight, wind up eating more calories while maintaining a lower weight than what was eaten to cause the excess weight in the first place. Proper nutrition can mean more calories with no weight gain, regardless of the rate of metabolism.

For anyone who might think they are an exception, that their metabolism is so slow that just about any small amount of food will cause weight gain, it cannot be true. The body, just to function, to breathe and get through the day, requires a certain amount of fuel, of calories. However low that amount might be for the person with the slowest metabolism, the amount of calories is not small. It still requires a certain amount of food with certain nutritional values eaten at regular enough intervals in a consistent enough manner to keep that body going. Even the slowest metabolism does not require anything near starvation. It still means food.

So, once a person loses the weight, the weight can be kept off.

The Metabolism Lady Story

I know a lady who went from thin to fat to thin, and in doing so accidentally solved the great metabolism issue all by herself. I met her when she was forty-one years old. She was nice, and she was about forty pounds overweight. She explained the excess weight by saying, "It is too bad I have such a slow metabolism. There is just nothing I can do about it." Of course, she was always on some sort of a diet, always talking about whatever diet she was on, and always gaining back whatever weight she lost on the diet after the diet ended, and then gaining a bit more weight beyond that. As a result, she continued to get heavier and more unhealthy.

Along came a day when I was in her house for a neighborhood gathering, and I saw an old picture of her. She looked so different I didn't recognize her. I had to diplomatically ask for clarification as to whether it was really her. In the picture she was twenty-eight years old and skinny. So I was now supposed to believe that not only was the cause of her weight problem a slow metabolism, but that the metabolism only became slow some time between the skinny picture and her current overweight point. Then one day she got skinny again.

It really took eight months, and here's what happened. She decided to begin eating right and exercising. I never did find out what the impetus was behind these dramatic changes, but I have heard of other people doing the same thing, i.e., not talking about the big changes. It is my belief that these people don't want to sound silly after going on so many diets, talking constantly about diets, then ultimately gaining weight as a direct result of dieting. I think they just wake up one day and a light goes on, and they see how ridiculous it all was. So silly that they can't fess up. They just shut up and start eating right and exercising. Real, proper eating. Fruits, vegetables, grains, no fat, and no pizza, donuts, burgers, fries, pies, or any other such junk. Only good things. Real movement too. Exercise. Our metabolism lady started doing aerobics and running, altogether eight to ten hours a week. After eight months of all this new, wonderful, positive stuff, she was back to the thin, healthy, ideal weight she had been at age twenty-eight.

Then one day she tripped and messed up her knee. She was helping a kindly, elderly man in a wheelchair cross a street. She was walking past him when she saw he needed some assistance. It was raining and the street and sidewalk were wet, and she slipped. An unusual accident, and such a little slip that she didn't even notice until the next morning when she couldn't get out of bed because her knee was swollen and throbbing. For three months she couldn't exercise, and her and her friends thought for sure she would get fat again. But guess what? She didn't gain an ounce. Nothing.

I could write a book on all she went through and all what happened, and the book would be this book. She grew up thin by eating pretty well and being fairly active. Then in her mid-twenties she started the raising-kids routine, which in the good life means junk food all the time, everywhere, and disastrous. Driving the kids to junk places. Pizza delivery. Not only did her kids and her kids' friends become overweight, but she did as well. Most of the other moms did too, and the dads. Metabolism had absolutely nothing to do with all these people gaining weight. The junk did. 100%. It's the food.

Now back to three months of no exercise after having become thin again and hurting her knee. How could she not gain weight?

It is seen elsewhere in this book that if a person is at his or her ideal weight (which is thin) and that person eats correctly, that person will stay at that ideal, thin, and healthy weight without exercise, and that is exactly what happened to our metabolism lady. After all she went through, I heard her say, with great difficulty, "It must not have been my metabolism after all. And the amazing thing is, I think I eat more now than I ever did before."

Of course she went back to exercising as soon as she could, because she had learned to love it and to understand all the many benefits. She didn't go back to the hours she had been doing when the light had gone on, but she didn't need to either. She was a happy woman.

The Exception

I am getting older, and I don't mean to be cruel, but so are you. Whatever age you are today, 29, 37, 45, 53, 66 or 109, you will be older tomorrow. I emphasize this, because no matter what age we are, as we get older our metabolism slows down. Every one of us. This is the exception to the "metabolism doesn't matter" statement. Once we hit the ripe young age of twenty-six or so, our bodies begin requiring less fuel, meaning our metabolism, rather fast, slow or in between, begins to slow down, so if we continue to eat and move at the same rates, we will gain weight. If this wasn't enough of a kicker, most every person on the face of the earth slows down physically as they get older. This is the only place where metabolism is relevant, and the message is clear. As soon as you can, meaning today, at whatever age and condition you are in, start eating correctly. Then read the chapter on exercise and follow the guidelines there to become an exerciser as soon as the program allows. The same theme, throughout, and here again, as a solution to this metabolism exception...

Eat Right and Exercise

...and even this aging thing can be dealt with.

The answer is always the same, and that is good news.

7

Exercise, Lexercise, and Butt-Sitting

Let's go. Move it. It's easy, really.

Not really. I had a tough time writing about this exercise thing, because:

> 1. Almost no one exercises, yet everyone knows they should.
>
> 2. Most people that try to get into an exercise routine stop within a few days of starting.
>
> 3. I have been an exerciser for thirty-two years.

So, what I am to do here, when exercise is easy for me but seemingly impossible for most people? I cannot be that much different, and I am lazy. The answer is: clarify things, because confusion reigns.

There is a vast amount of information that has been available for years about exercise. Way too much actually, like information on dieting. Unlike dieting info where about 98.27% is bad, misleading, or even harmful, most of what we have seen about exercise is true. But it is also difficult to err in regards to exercise, since about all you need to know is that it is good for you, and everyone already knows that. Most everyone also knows what it means to exercise. Move. Work up a sweat. But for various reasons almost no one exercises. Since everyone knows they should exercise, but almost no one does, we need to find out why.

Since I am trying to make this book different from other books that deal with exercise, I won't do the usual, which is to tell all about why we should exercise and then give the traditional exercise advice. The implication from this regular-advice-format is that all we have to do is explain why we should exercise, then list the exercises, and then everyone is expected to go off to start huffing, puffing, and sweating. Since most people don't exercise, though, and everyone is familiar with the drill, the drill must not work. We are going to take a different track then, to get moving.

But first a note about who exercises and who doesn't. I have seen numerous reports that claim that as much as 30% to the even more ridiculous number of 65% of adults exercise, and neither of these figures is even close. They are way too high. When I wrote that almost no one exercises, that is exactly what I mean. I believe the real percentage of people that exercise is more like 3%, and on the outside, 8%. So when you do go about moving about, for the most part when you see someone else exercising, you will be seeing a familiar face. There are only a few of us out there. You and me and a couple others. Now another digression.

Exercisers Are Wonderful People

Exercisers are among the nicest people in the world. Most everyone that I know who exercises (and please refer to the upcoming definition of what exercise means, because along with other things, it does not mean weight lifting or "blading") is a nice person. Isn't that amazing? If it holds true, and you become an exerciser, you will be a wonderful, nice person, even if you aren't now. And if you aren't now, what a terrific thing to look forward to.

Which makes me wonderful and nice, it would seem. But I don't mean to brag. I just want to give you another reason to exercise: to meet nice people. When I was in my early thirties, I moved to Beaverton, Oregon, a suburb of Portland. By that time I had been a runner for twelve years. Once in Beaverton I developed a desire to run a marathon. Ours was a new neighborhood with most homes occupied by couples around the same age as my wife and I. Some people were seen running, and eventually I hooked up with a few of these folks, and they were nice. Then more people started running together, and then things started to get organized. I made an attempt to set a schedule so that people knew at what time the group would be running, from whose house on what days. The "whose house" didn't change though, because our house happened to be the last one we would pass on the way out of the subdivision. Every day for the remaining year and a half that we lived there, runners met at our house. Maybe one or two or none on some days, but on Sunday mornings often as many as thirteen. Early on Sundays most everyone was available, and some people came who only did such moving around once a week. The people would divide into two groups, with the more serious runners going off in one direction and the less serious going in another. Usually everyone would meet when done and visit a bit, and every few months the talk would turn into brunch planning, and an hour later dozens of people would be gathered having fun. The neighborhood grew ever closer, friends were made, and a lot of everyone's social lives revolved around that group of exercisers. Great times, great fun, and memories to last a lifetime. And everyone was wonderful. So there might be more to look forward to than what first meets the mind.

What Is Exercise?

Most fitness instructors and experts have pretty much agreed for a long time that exercise is physical activity that gets the heart rate up to a certain level and keeps it at that rate for at least 20 minutes, and which is done 3 to 4 times per week. While I agree for the most part, it is just that kind of information that causes people to quit their new exercise program right after they start it, or worse, before they even begin. So forget the normal advice. No one who has not exercised in decades, or who has never exercised, can exercise for 20 minutes. And what is this magical heart rate level thing? What are you supposed to do that first day? Questions and confusion. (We will get back to the heart rate thing later in this chapter.) A friend of mine once decided he was going to become a runner, so he told me he was going to start running with me, and that to start, he was going to run "just three miles." You know, start easy. He made it 1/8th of a mile. Reality hit him. Let's you and I hit reality first by forgetting the common and finding a way that will work. A different approach. Not the old drill.

There is a matter regarding this search for exercise that is a most critical one, and it is one most people do that insures failure and that coincides with the 20 minute guideline mentioned above. They set goals that are not attainable. Expectations are so high that it is impossible to be successful. People learn quickly that they can only fail, so they quit. Since most people don't exercise and never have exercised, the idea of starting from a point of nothing and getting to a high level of physical activity in a short period of time is impossible. Failure is guaranteed. So the first thing we are going to do is not do something. Don't set goals. You will have a plan, though, and it will basically just call for you to move. Just move.

The first part of the plan is to start. Choose what exercise you are going to do (some suggestions will be made shortly) and begin moving. Slowly and easily. Not fast or long. Just be comfortable. It won't matter if you only go for three minutes or ten or whatever. Remember, most people, and maybe you, not only do not exercise, but have never exercised. The moving around we did as kids was just play, or sports, and I don't consider organized athletics in high school or even college as exercise, because, to the definition of exercise I add that we exercise "for our health and well-being." We do not exercise to burn calories.

Did you see that? We do not exercise to burn calories. While most people think that is why we exercise, and most books, articles and programs about exercise say we exercise to burn calories, we don't. At least you won't. I know I don't. It just doesn't make sense. If the only reason we exercise is to burn off excess calories, why not just stop eating the excess calories? If a person is not overweight and eats right, then that person will remain thin without exercising, so he or she doesn't need to exercise if we use this burning-calorie rule. On the other hand, if a person is overweight now, then starts eating right and exercising and as a result loses all the excess weight, that person can then stop exercising. This takes us back to the question "Why exercise?" and we come to the same answer: because it is good for us. You are not trying to do X amount of exercise, X amount of days, for X months, to lose X pounds, and then quit. You are going to exercise because it is good for you, and a side benefit will be that if you are overweight, exercise will help you to lose weight as you simultaneously begin eating correctly. When the excess weight is lost, you will keep exercising, because it is good for you. So, no goals. You just need to start, and hopefully it will be easier to do that now that you won't be doing it for the wrong reason.

You Can't Run It Off

Sometimes I harp, and I am such a fervent believer in the value of exercise that I want as many people exercising as possible. But people need to go about it properly, by not setting goals that can't be reached, by starting easily and slowly, and also by being realistic about not only what exercise can do for them, but also by understanding what it cannot do. This is not to discourage people, but rather to help have as broad an understanding as possible in order to maximize our efforts. So I am harping here about goals, and therefore the bold statement above that says "You Can't Run It Off."

One of the strongest beliefs about exercise is that if you exercise enough, no matter how overweight you are, you will become thin. You can work it off, run it off, sweat it off, or huff-and-puff it off. But it just isn't true, and that reality comes from the following: a person who is overweight and who has never exercised cannot exercise enough to burn off all the fat. It just takes too much effort. To lose one pound requires exercising enough to "burn" off 3500 calories. Running is one of the most efficient forms of calorie-burning exercises, and since running one mile burns off only one hundred calories, it would take thirty-five miles of running to lose one pound. So, three hundred fifty miles to lose ten pounds, and there is almost no one that is only ten pounds overweight. I once heard a person say, "I need to lose about fifteen or twenty pounds," but I can assure you that person needed to lose thirty just to not look fat, and fifty to be thin. Most adults who have not just fallen off the turnip truck, who have never exercised and who have been eating incorrectly their whole life, are at least twenty pounds overweight, so for these people, it would take seven hundred miles of running to get rid of the extra twenty pounds. So, never exercised, out of shape with partially clogged arteries, elevated cholesterol, and overweight, and now that person is going to go run seven hundred miles? It just can't be done. It won't be done. Over what period of time? Not many "experts" I have come across mention time. Over what period of time does the person have to run the seven hundred miles? A month? Of course not, and not in six months either. What about people who need to lose forty pounds (and there are plenty of those)? They would have to run fourteen hundred miles. Just more silly stuff, as I hope is becoming obvious. It just can't be done. How is the overweight, out-of-shape person going to run three hundred fifty to fourteen hundred miles? Forget how, and don't set unattainable goals. The only way to reverse the damage our lifestyle has caused is to eat right and exercise. So, one stone is overturned: you can't run it off, so don't try to run it off or work it off, or burn it off, or sweat it off, because if you try you will give up and quit, probably forever. Just begin moving, once you get the rest of the directions on how to do so, and start eating correctly.

Digression

There was one fellow I did observe who was quite overweight who did exercise it off. I saw him go from fat to thin, a number of times. It was remarkable to watch. The cycle went like this: once he got about sixty pounds overweight by eating horribly, he would virtually stop eating and simultaneously begin a very grueling exercise program. Six or seven days a week he would exercise, for two to three hours at a time. In the hour prior to each exercise session, he would drink a gallon of water, so during each workout he would become soaking wet. He exerted himself to unbelievable levels almost every day for months. He would lose all the extra pounds, actually look skinny, relative to his obese days, then stop exercising completely, start eating terribly again, gain the sixty pounds back, and back and forth. So in truth, a person can exercise it off, but the effort required is so huge that it is virtually impossible.

I am also familiar with people who are very overweight who exercise a lot and yet remain overweight. I have watched some of them run four to five times a week for thirty to fifty minutes at a time for years and remain the same large size as the first time I saw them. We can assume a couple things here: first, that they are healthier than if they didn't run, and secondly, that they eat so badly that there is literally no amount of exercise that will make them thin. It seems like such a waste, because the only reason they are doing all that running is to lose weight, but the weight loss never happens. Perhaps they would gain an additional forty pounds or so if they stopped the running, but since so much time, effort, and energy is involved, why wouldn't they take some of that and direct it towards better eating habits? Anyway, more proof to me that "you can't run it off."

For you skeptics, I am forced to add a not-so-pleasant story here. There are those reading this who will say, "Of course I can run it off," and go off thinking they know everything. They won't go off to exercise, but if they did, they would be thinking that all their excess weight would soon go away. Let's look at someone who, sadly, did run it off, while still eating poorly.

One day I was at my local community recreation center talking to someone about this book, and a woman in her mid-fifties overheard and politely interrupted, so she could tell her story. She was not there at the rec center to exercise, but rather to watch her husband, who was fifty-seven years old, exercise, and this woman was visibly distressed. Her husband was a runner, and he was thin. When he ran, he would run three miles. After his runs, he would eat two cheeseburgers, french fries, and a milk shake. Then he had a heart attack and nearly died. The wife was anguished, because the husband was in denial. He thought he shouldn't have had a heart attack because he exercised, while all the wife knew was that the next heart attack would likely be fatal. She didn't know what to do, and it was sad. It might be said that he "ran it off," that he exercised enough to be thin, but the running could not offset the bad eating. The excess calories did indeed get "burned off," but his arteries were clogged from the excess fat. So don't fool yourself, because you can't fool nature.

Moving On

By this time I hope we all agree on the following:

A. Exercise is good for us. (It's great, actually.)

B. Do not set unrealistic goals.

C. Don't try to use exercise alone as your way to weight loss and improved health. Just start moving slowly and regularly, and start eating right. Good things will follow, and you will become healthy, fit, and thin.

Now, in regards to the moving part.

Whatever exercise you are going to do, you will want to do it slowly and easily, especially in the beginning. Slow and easy is the plan.

Before you start moving, though, let's take a look at various types of exercise to help you determine what you are going to undertake. I have heard a saying about exercise that goes something like this: "The best exercise is the one you will do." While this is true, there are some issues regarding efficiency and effectiveness that need to be looked at to help ensure on-going success. One is that since you will need to get your heart rate up, the best and easiest way to do that is to use those large muscle groups below your waist: your legs, thighs, and butt, and such. Whatever exercise you undertake, then, you need to be on your feet. Like walking, running, treadmills, step machines, aerobics, and so forth. Doing things short of being on your feet, like stationary biking, make it difficult to get the heart rate up high enough to get the types of benefits you need. This is good news though, because the type of activity I recommend starting with is familiar and easy. Walking. What could be easier? Just start walking, whether in the neighborhood, around a track indoors or outdoors, or on a treadmill. Wherever. Move faster than a stroll on the beach with a loved one, but not so fast that you look like a nut, get fatigued, and have to stop. Since you are about to become an official exerciser, go get some good shoes, dress like a real, official exerciser (the dress code is upcoming), and move.

Two Things Now…Your Doctor and Looking Pretty

I have an obligation and a responsibility to tell the readers of this book that before they embark on a new exercise program they should see a doctor and get a complete physical examination. In fact, this is the second time I have written this. The medical exam is a must. When I turned 40, I had a complete physical, even though I had been eating better than average for 10 years, and even though I had been running for nearly 20, and even though I was thin. I still did it, and you need to do it. We are not trying to be heroes here, so we can slow down, see the doctor, get the physical, and then start moving.

Being pretty. Every year in the days that follow Christmas, the regular runners at the recreation center where I used to run would watch with amusement as the wanna-be's would show up for their first ever in their lifetime exercise session wearing pretty, fancy, colorful, and stylish new athletic wear, obviously given to them as Christmas presents. This year, for sure, they are going to start exercising. Real runners and real exercisers aren't stylish. Get some plain sweats, good shoes, and get moving. You don't have to be stylish. By the way, we used to put bets on how long it would be before the people with the pretty new clothes would stop coming. Most of the pretty ones we would see just once, and by mid-January they would all be gone.

Things That Aren't Exercise

There are certain types of physical activity that people might consider doing, but according to the definition of exercise, and/or from a safety perspective, they don't qualify as exercise. You won't do them as exercise, but rather just for fun, for recreation, if you do them at all. Please don't be alarmed if something you might be thinking of doing is on my not-to-do list. There are plenty of other choices, as we will get too.

Looking at the don'ts:

1. <u>Biking</u>

The main thing here is the danger of getting hurt. The probability of falling off the bike and getting hurt is nearly 100%. Getting your heart rate up to where you want it requires too high of a speed, and it is speed that will surely cause a fall. Also, depending on where you live, there could be far too many days when inclement weather will prevent riding anyway. There is too much stacked against biking.

2. <u>In-line skating (or "blading" as some like to call it)</u>

I have never tried in-line skating, but it looks like a blast. I skated hundreds and maybe thousands of miles when I was a kid, on steel-wheeled, old-fashion skates, and had a ton of fun. There is a problem with skating though, when it comes to exercise. It is very difficult to get your heart rate up high enough, and it is especially hard to maintain such a high speed for the length of time required. Incidentally, you also have the issues of falling and getting hurt, of bad weather preventing exercise, and of finding a decent place to skate.

I pause, for those of you who have seen what appears to be the obvious, but isn't. I have seen it also, and I might very well have seen more of it than most, because I spend so much time running outdoors in nice weather along the beautiful lakefront in Chicago. I am talking about the fantastic looking, athletic looking, body-perfect, tanned, gorgeous women gliding smoothly along on in-line skates. There is something very sexy about women who fit the description just offered, especially when they are in nothing more than a bikini or some other such slim attire. The guys who fit the description just detailed look good also, I guess, so the innocent observer might very well conclude that in-line skating is the only way to go. Of all the people exercising, these are the only ones that look that good. But they aren't really exercising anyway. They're just "blading." And trust me, none of these people got that look by way of in-line skating. First, they were born with good looks, then they became athletic through hard physical exercise, and finally, they did a lot of intense tanning. Major league, time-consuming tanning. The in-line skating is used by such people as a fun, show-offy activity. So as good as they look, just look and get on with some real exercise.

3. Swimming

Swimming is not what you are going to do either. It is hard to get your heart rate up high enough, because it is not done on the feet.

4. Stationary biking

The problem here is also that of not being able to get your heart rate up to the level you want. It can be done, but the effort required does not make this form of exercise viable. The stationary bike can, however, come into play in a couple situations. First, when you are just beginning your new exercise program and you are going slowly and easily, the bike can work well. Once your program develops to a higher level, the bike will have to go, except for maybe a day or two a week when you want to exercise but at a reduced level.

The other place for the stationary bike is if and when you might have a slight injury from running or whatever, and rather than not exercise at all while healing, a stationary bike might at least keep you active.

5. <u>Walking or running with weights</u>

I see people walking and running for exercise while they are carrying hand weights and/or have weights attached to their ankles and/or waist. The incremental value of these weights is near or at zero, but the extra work could discourage you from exercising at all. Forget the weights and relax while you move.

6. <u>Tennis now and then</u>

Most people that play tennis don't do it hard enough or do it long enough for it to be called exercise. Look at tennis as a recreational activity and have fun when you play it.

7. <u>Golf</u>

I am a golfer, and I love golf, and I don't want to get into a debate with any of my golfing friends concerning whether or not golf is exercise. But, being objective and looking back at the definition of exercise answers the question. It isn't. But it sure is a fun game, and it can wear you out, and it takes a lot of energy, and you can sweat a lot, but there it ends. We are trying to get healthy, fit, and thin, so let's not fool ourselves.

I have a painting that shows a golfer in mid-swing. The golfer is wearing a tie. Granted the image is from the old days when golfers wore ties, but the point is, there is no exercise that would ever require the wearing of a tie. Not in the old days, not today, and not tomorrow.

8. <u>Bowling</u>

Not even close. This is way behind golf, and this is not a knock on bowling or bowlers. I love bowlers, too. In fact, just the other day I kissed a beautiful lady who was bowling. (It was my wife.)

9. <u>Strolling</u>

A walk after dinner once in a while or a stroll here and there from time to time, is not exercise. It can be relaxing and enjoyable, but it is not going to help turn things around. I stroll a lot, especially after a run, but I don't put that in my exercise log as exercise.

Moving On To Moving

Now get going. Since we saw that we want to be on our feet, I suggest you start by walking, and then move up to something else later, like running, aerobics, step machines or whatever. Start with walking, because it is so easy and natural. Get someone to go with you if at all possible (see Chapter 11, Pretty Pink Bra...i.e., Get Some Support), pick a route and walk. Move just a bit faster than a normal walk. Enjoy, and then do it on as many days as possible, at least in the beginning. Ten minutes, fifteen, twenty, whatever. The idea is to get into the habit of moving, a regular routine, comfortable, and build up from there. I offer the following formula to show how this all comes together:

START

and

START SLOWLY

and

STICK WITH IT

while

GRADUALLY DOING MORE

until

YOU GET IN SHAPE

then
KEEP GOING
until
IT BECOMES A HABIT
or
EASY
or
"LIKE BRUSHING MY TEETH"

During a visit to a health club one cold Chicago winter day, I noticed a woman moving very aggressively on a step machine. I first saw her when I was getting ready to run, and when I finished running I saw that she was still going. Once I had walked around for a while and cooled down, she finally stopped. She must have been on that machine for an hour and a half. I wanted to know what her deal was, so I went to talk to her. At the conclusion of her explanation of her exercise program, she said that it had become easy, "like brushing my teeth." It does become easy.

So you are going to start, and start slowly, and you are going to stick with it, not because of some rah, rah coming from this book or from any other source, but as a result of taking a different approach, and you are going to succeed.

I am not going to even suggest a schedule to follow to build up to the level you will eventually want to reach, but keep in mind that part of the definition of exercise says to get your heart rate up to a certain level and leave it there for twenty minutes minimum, three to four times per week. The important thing is to get to where, at some comfortable point in time, you are exercising twenty minutes at a time. Take as long as you want to get there. Once you are there you can begin working on increasing your speed to get your heart rate up higher. Since you will be monitoring your heart rate, let's look at the formula for measuring it. This measuring is not exact science, however. You will use it just as a guideline and let common sense, experience, your doctor, and how you feel all contribute to the intensity and length of your exercise sessions.

The heart rate guide is easy to use once you learn it and work with it for a while. You start by determining your maximum heart rate, which is the number 220 minus your age. So, if you are forty years old your maximum heart rate is 180 beats per minute. You will want to get your heart rate up to about 40% to 60% of your maximum and keep it there for the twenty minutes we have been talking about. There is no rush, so take as long as you need. (Even a slow walk might get your heart rate up to those levels in the beginning of your new exercise program.) Again, this is not exact science. Your doctor will give you some guidelines. Just pay attention to what is going on. By that I mean when you first start exercising and you walk slowly, note your heart rate. If it is in the 40% to 60% range and you feel good and within that range is where your doctor says you should be, and that rate is about the same each time you walk, you are doing fine. Don't try to complicate things. You should see consistent numbers and be comfortable and feel good. As you move faster and longer the rates should go up. If you continue at a slow walk for a long time, like months, your heart rate might actually begin to go down as a result of getting your heart and body in better condition. So listen to your head and see how you feel, and enjoy. Build up over time, at your own pace. We talked about not setting unrealistic goals, but these goals of 40% to 60% and twenty minutes at a time are easily obtainable. As long as you start eating right and move frequently, you will be able to get to where you want to be. To check your rate just hold your finger against the large artery in your neck and count how many beats there are in fifteen seconds, then multiply that by four.

A little more is in order about this heart rate thing. The 40% to 60% rates mentioned above are beginning levels for those people who are in the early phase of a new exercise program, and target heart rates go up from there. Down the road, you will want to get your heart rate up to 70%, and if you really get into this exercise thing and train for a running event, you might train as high as 80%. So 70% to 80% is where you might expect to be after you become a real, on-going, in shape, thin, experienced exerciser. Way down the road.

In the beginning, you will want to play it safe, watch your pulse, and know where your heart rate is at all times. If your heart rate is going a lot faster than it should, you should stop until the rate goes down. Once you get in shape, are thin, and your doctor gives you the OK, you can then start moving the heart rate up with more vigorous exercise. Later though.

The 20/20 Club…In Other Words, Look At What 40 Can Do

I want to mention something here that in no way pertains to today or tomorrow, but down the road. You might call it a goal, but I won't because I am being defensive. I will call it a "long-term objective" or a "nice thing to do at some time in the future." It has to do with the length of time that you exercise. I read somewhere, many years ago, that the first 20 minutes is for the body and the second 20 minutes is for the head. The first 20 corresponds to all we have seen in this book and elsewhere about the need to exercise for 20 minutes whenever you exercise (once you are able to build up to the level, no matter how long it takes). But I found out long ago during my own exercising that the 20 plus 20 thing is true. Once you have been moving for a while, around 20 minutes or so, the body and the mind begin to relax, and the exercise becomes effortless, and the second 20 minutes goes quickly and is the real fun part. Not that the first 20 is hard, because you will get to a point where it isn't, but obviously starting out you have to get going, get into the pace, warm up and all. It is during the second 20 minutes that I really start to feel good both physically and mentally, solve problems, get creative, think positively, and get fired up about life. That is why whenever I get done running, I am psyched, and I see this with about everyone who exercises. So down the road, give the 20/20 thing a try.

Don't Work Out

The term "workout" is used by most people to describe exercise, but you will not "work out," so your exercise will never be called a "workout." You will not be working at this. It is not work, and if you ever get to a point where your exercise is strenuous enough to perhaps be called work, that will be a long time from now, well into a regular program when you have become healthy, fit, and thin and you are officially training for an athletic event. So, for now and way down the road, and maybe forever, don't "work out," just relax, go slowly and enjoy. Real exercisers, people who have been exercising regularly for years, don't work out, because it is not difficult, so it can't be work. Like runners. I am one, and I run for my head, and the physical benefits follow. I love running, and it requires virtually no effort, and you will get to that point too, in time. I don't work out. I run.

Lexercise

As mentioned earlier, there has been a lot of bad information spread around about exercise. Some of the bad stuff comes from people who believe that little pieces of exercise add up to real exercise, but that just isn't true for us. On the surface it might seem to hold, but the theory doesn't work for our purposes. People even add up activity such as walking from the couch to the television to change stations rather than using the remote control as contributing to exercise goals. The real benefits of exercise come from exercise that is continuous, that gets the heart rate up, and which will eventually grow to 20 minutes or longer, 3 to 4 times a week.

For people who have spent a lifetime eating badly and never exercising, and as a result having their arteries get clogged up, becoming overweight, and putting themselves at risk for all kinds of lifestyle related diseases and illnesses, it takes major changes to make things better. The notion that there are shortcuts only decreases the probability of success. Don't pay any attention to the idea that things like using the stairs instead of the elevator and parking farther away from where you are going will count as exercise, burn calories, and make you healthy, fit, and thin. Instead, do whatever is possible in order to save up enough time to do some real exercise. The word "lexercise" I made up, and it derives from the words "less than exercise." There is no such thing, and therefore it has no meaning and no value. The "little bits" mean nothing to you.

Butt-sitting

I didn't make up the term butt-sitting. Far too many people have been doing it way too much for far too long for me to take credit for the term. I do encourage people to do a lot less of it, though, so they can spend time exercising. For most people, all the time needed to exercise, plus a whole lot more, can be found by simply turning the TV off. Watching TV is by far the most useless of butt-sitting activities ever undertaken by mankind. So butt-sitting can end today. Hit the "OFF" button.

The hours wasted. The life gone. If the typical person, who as we saw earlier watches 1,000 hours of TV a year, was to turn the doodad off and exercise instead, an amazing thing would happen. In just five short years they would lose 850 pounds and be much healthier. (We saw earlier that the calories in/calories out formula doesn't really work, but the fact remains, a lot less TV would be good for all the people all the time.)

Back to the Beginning

In the beginning of this chapter, I chose to not detail reasons we should exercise. But I can't leave it at that, because understanding the value of exercise is just too big of a deal. Hopefully by leaving it until the end like this, you will be better able to start on an exercise program, because it will have more meaning. Because your confidence level will be higher. Let's look, now, at some of the things exercise can do. It can:

1. Relieve stress, both mental and physical.

2. Reduce the risk of developing diabetes.

3. Reduce the risk of developing high blood pressure.

4. Reduce the risk of developing colon cancer.

5. Reduce the chance of dying prematurely from heart disease.

6. Help control weight.

7. Help to alleviate depression.

8. Improve the functioning of the body's immune system.

9. Increase energy.

10. Help to make bones healthy and thereby delay or prevent osteoporosis.

11. Improve the quality of life.

12. Help you live longer.

I could keep going, and in fact I have in front of me a poster that has "101 Reasons to Exercise," but I trust you know enough now anyway, and besides, you probably want to quit reading and get going.

Not yet, though. Just a few more things. As soon as you start exercising, the first time you do anything, you will feel the effect, because you will feel good about yourself. In the head. More good news.

Ouch

"I don't run, because running is bad for the knees," said the fat guy while eating a double cheeseburger with fries and a shake.

"What exercise do you do then?" asked Gary.

"None."

Bad information shows up even regarding injury, not unlike the dialogue just seen. It is surprising how many people believe that running is bad on the knees. But I have not seen a study that supports this concern. My conclusion, then, is that running does not lead to injuries. More to the point, caution about injuries from any type of exercise should not focus on any particular potential problem, but rather on the general approach that could lead to an unwanted setback. If a person has not exercised for a long time, that person will be subject to injury if he or she is too aggressive by trying to do too much or by going too fast. A person has to start easily, or of course problems can arise. When we were kids running and jumping and such, we virtually never got hurt and getting sore was impossible. But as we get older we are much more susceptible to injury. It's just a fact of life, and that is why I have gone to lengths earlier in this chapter to emphasize that the only way to begin an exercise program is to do it slowly and easily.

It should go without saying, but I will say it anyway. If a person has excess weight, the probability of injury is increased. Easy please, so you can keep moving. I work with people one-on-one to help them become healthy, fit, and thin, and whenever I start working with a new client and we get to the exercise part, talk about it, and start planning it, I ask what length of time and at what speed the client intends to begin. 100% of the clients state speed and time levels that are way too high. Getting healthy, fit, and thin takes time, whatever time that is. There is no deadline, and as a great Nike poster says, "There is no finish line™." There is no hurry, it is gradual, and there is every reason in the world to not force things.

Take it easy and build up, develop new habits, clear your head, get healthy, start losing weight, feel better and look better, all at a pace that will allow you to continue. Forever.

Tips and Suggestions

I know you are anxious to get moving, so I will hit just briefly on a few more areas that I think are important.

1. Don't run on grass

It is too easy to twist an ankle or a knee, because while the grass might look smooth, the ground under it might not be. I cringe at some of the injuries I've seen and heard about as a result of people running or playing on grass. Spare me any more stories and "keep off the grass."

2. Don't warm up before exercise

We have all probably heard that we should warm up before exercise, but for most of us here, it isn't necessary. We are going to be moving so slowly and easily, that there will be nothing to warm up for. We can save some time then. Just begin your exercise at a slow pace and increase as you go along. Technically, doing so is "warming up." When you get to a higher level of exercise, fine, but I have yet to "warm up." And I am in my 33rd year of running.

3. Do warm down

Take it easy right after you exercise. If, immediately upon ending your exercise, you were to stop all movement, you could have a problem. Walk around a bit, relax, keep moving, slowly, and let your heart rate move down gradually.

4. Frequency again

The common advice about how often to exercise is 3 to 4 times a week, and I agree. However, in the beginning, when a person has never exercised and is trying to develop new, lifelong, positive habits and the exercise is slow and easy and not all that long in duration, I suggest exercising as many days as possible. Why not every day?

5. <u>Spot reducing</u>

There is no such thing. Once you become healthy, fit, and thin, the question won't matter anyway.

Magic

It is mentioned throughout this book that there is no such thing as magic or miracles, but look at what Dr. JoAnn Manson, chief of preventive medicine at Harvard's Brigham and Women's Hospital said: "Regular physical activity is probably as close to a magic bullet as we will come in modern medicine." (Time Magazine, 1-2-02). So move it.

8

Stretching

Stretch what? Why? Don't bother.

I am in my 33rd year of running. I have averaged 3.2 days of running per week, which means I have run over 5,300 times, and the number of times I have stretched prior to a run is zero. For all practical purposes, I have had no injuries. But most of the thousands of books and articles on exercising say to stretch, and, as you might expect, there are numerous books dedicated just to stretching. So, you have something like 99.45% of all exercise advisors telling you to stretch, and lonely me saying it's not necessary, so what are you to do?

Before deciding, let's remember what we are trying to do here. We have recognized that almost no one exercises and that one of the main excuses is time. While I personally don't think a lack of time should be an issue, because exercise is fun and exercise creates time due to creating energy, I am trying to help. I am also being realistic. So let's concede for the present that stretching takes time that you don't have. And since you have at least one person, me, telling you that you don't need to stretch, use that for an excuse, don't stretch, and save the time. With that said, the discussion can end right here. But let me expand a bit, to give you a specific reason not to stretch. Something besides, "You don't need to stretch."

You are not in training for an athletic competition. All this stuff is probably new, the eating right and exercising. As the chapter on exercise points out, you are going to start slowly and easily. You will probably start with a little walking. As a result, stretching muscles that are not going to do anything other than walk slowly just isn't necessary. That's it.

By the way, you can actually pull a muscle stretching if you have never stretched, are out of shape, and don't know how to stretch properly. So now you have two specific reasons to not stretch. I'm just full of good news.

Now, my catch-all. I am not saying "don't ever stretch." Stretching is a part of total fitness, in the long run. And, it is almost a must as you get more aggressive in your exercise program. When the walking turns into slow jogging that turns into running. Once you get your overall program going, the eating right and exercising. But there is no rush. Some day, down the road, you should begin to stretch. When you do, learn how to do it properly to both minimize the chances of pulling a muscle and to maximize whatever benefits can be obtained. Just take it easy. My point is that you don't need to spend the time right now if time is a concern.

9

Ladies, Please

This chapter is offered to a special group of people, one that I am particularly fond of. (But the guys can read it also.)

Nature and society, being what they are, place more emphasis on a woman's appearance than they do a man's. If a woman is just 10% overweight, she might be referred to in negative terms, and she might think of herself in the same manner. If a man has the same weight situation, or if he is even more overweight than the woman just described, he might actually be referred to in positive terms such as "husky" or "muscular." Women react to the extra weight by going on diets much more frequently than men. If this was the end of it, meaning that if women went on diets, lost weight, got back to normal, and stayed there, it would be bad enough, because dieting causes so much grief. But it is not the end, because diets don't work. In fact, it is at this point where the situation gets considerably worse and slams into even more serious problems, such as:

1. Constant long-term weight gain: Since dieting actually causes weight gain over time, overweight women continue to get heavier, thereby adding to the poor self-image and negative social consequences excess weight can cause.

2. Increases in potential health problems: Since many serious health conditions are caused and/or aggravated by excess weight, overweight women keep getting more unhealthy.

Women need to move beyond the focus of weight to the broader, more important areas of overall health and fitness. Thinness will follow. To support such a plan, I refer to an article written by Liz Grapentine titled "Women & Heart Disease" (Healthy Woman Magazine): "only eight percent of American women consider heart disease and stroke to be their greatest health threats. In fact, cardiovascular disease claims more female lives every year than the next 16 causes of death combined and nearly twice as many as do all forms of cancer."

So, ladies, please, join me in trying to learn what we can do to make things better. Focus on your health and well-being, and you will become healthy, fit, and thin. Discard the ridiculous that has been forced on us all and explore solutions. Stop making the diet companies rich, and instead start becoming the person you want to be and can be. Not just not overweight, but healthy, positive, and active. So you can enjoy your success and the good life.

Extra Good News For Women Only

It was noted above that women go on diets a lot more than men. That is understandable, with all the pressures to be thin and all the diet promises. Hopefully, though, this book will help women to see the fallacy of dieting. But the diet thing is not the end for the fairer sex. Some how, over time, women have been lead down a few other dead ends. Perhaps identifying some will help. Like these:

> I frequently see women exercise by walking rapidly with their arms literally flailing away. The incremental benefit of doing this is about zero, so I don't understand it. I think that somewhere along the line someone tried to sell women on the idea that flapping their arms wildly while walking would help them lose weight, but doing the arm thing absolutely doesn't help lose weight, and it looks silly. Add those facts to the fact that we don't exercise to lose weight anyway, and the flailing can end. This wouldn't be a big deal with me, certainly not to where I would include it in this

book, if it wasn't for the fact that it is only women who do it. If I have seen 3,584 women do it, I have seen just one man, and that was so unusual it startled me. I saw him out of the corner of my eye while I was running recently, and my first thought was, "What in the heck is he doing," when it hit me that I had never seen a man do that. So ladies, give it up, because it must just come from someone trying to sell women something useless. That's my point. Worthless information. Please don't be a target for nonsense.

> Many women run on their toes. I'm pretty sure this is just a function of being female, because virtually no males do it. It probably doesn't come from someone trying to pass bad information. Either way, it can cause injury, so for those women who run on their toes, please take the effort to run the other way. When a foot comes down to meet the ground, the heel needs to touch first, then the foot rolls forward, and you then push off with the front of the foot.

> It is my observation that there are too many women who walk and run for exercise who do so with hand and/or ankle weights. Probably more women than men, leading me to believe, again, that bad information has been disproportionately aimed at women. And women bought this too. Since, as far as I am concerned, the hand and ankle weights serve no purpose, don't bother. Forget the hassle, just relax, and go.

Extra good news? I think so, because with the right news, success can follow.

10

Why Do Overweight People Lift Weights To Lose Weight?

More than ever, it seems that when health and fitness are being discussed, the need to lift weights is thrown into the mix, as if pumping iron will make a person healthy, fit, and thin. So we now see overweight people lifting weights to lose weight, and I think this is ridiculous.

The craziness goes like this: since muscle burns calories, and a person needs to burn calories to lose weight, a person needs to lift weights to build more muscle so they will have more muscle to burn more calories. I just hate to see people be responsive to this idea. But more and more they are. They start a physical fitness program, something they have probably never done before, and go through all the time, discipline, sweat, energy expenditure and such, to develop larger muscles. Therefore, they will become heavier, so they can burn more calories because they have more muscles, because they are overweight. Talk about convoluted.

We need to return to square one here. If you are overweight and you want to begin to make changes for the better, focus on the sound and the simple. Eat right and exercise.

Female Bones

I'm sure most women know that strength training is a good thing, and it is. It can increase bone density which can help prevent or delay osteoporosis. We read about this all the time. (Osteoporosis is brittle bones that is common among older people, especially women, and can lead to serious problems.) I need to note that I am not downplaying the importance of this benefit of pumping iron, but I have to fall back on my original premise. People need to start eating right and exercising to reverse the damages caused by the good life and to begin getting healthy, fit, and thin. When those things are significantly, properly, and successfully put in place, incorporating strength training into their program should be done. I want women to lift weights, and when I work with women individually, I insist on it. After a while. The women have to first start with eating right and exercising. Then, when progress towards their overall goals is seen, lifting weights begin. The iron will then be pumped for the right reason.

(This all pertains to men also, because total fitness involves strength training. But the weights wait until a person gets fit and then starts making efforts to become totally fit.)

11

Pretty Pink Bra...i.e., Get Some Support

One day, long ago, I decided I wanted to run a marathon. A marathon is 26.2 miles, and as I can now say (after having run not one, but two marathons), don't worry about the .2 at the end. Just watch out for the first 26. Those are the ones that can hurt, and cause second thoughts, loneliness, blisters, muscles cramps, and fear. However, none of those is the topic here, nor is it even the running of a marathon. Rather, I want to talk about the aspect of exercise that deals with the actual doing it part. The getting-it-done thing. (I'll do some of it via marathoning, though, because I think the analogy is relevant.)

Some people reflect on the thought of running a marathon by asking, "Why would you do that?" To me, though, the pertinent question should be, "Why in the world would you do that alone?" There is such a tremendously large amount of training and related effort required in order to even attempt a marathon. The miles alone are overwhelming enough to cause most people to give up early in a training program or, of course, to never consider such an undertaking in the first place. It's work and time, and it takes six months to prepare to run a marathon if a person is already a runner, and up to a year if a person goes into the training without already being a runner. What if you have a spouse and you are taking time away from that person and maybe kids too, and missing dinner, and your spouse is groaning? There was a guy in the neighborhood I lived in during my marathon days who had done the training for a marathon the year prior to my doing so, and when I made the suggestion that he join the group I was training with, his wife responded by saying, "Gary, if he does that again I will divorce him and kill you!" I didn't pursue his assistance any further.

The point is, it can be difficult to accomplish certain goals, like exercise goals, if we do it alone. Most people who begin an exercise program do it by themselves, and they fail to continue for any length of time. But there is plenty of evidence that doing things with other people can help a person stick with a program. As Bob Condor, a staff writer for the Chicago Tribune, reported in one of his "Training Table" articles, "Exercising with a partner is an equally good idea for your fitness program. The biggest advantage is motivation; if you are obligated to meet someone for a tennis match or to walk a few miles together to catch up on gossip, chances are you won't cancel."

It would seem obvious that getting someone to help you start and stay with an exercise program would increase the chance of success, but most people still go about it alone, probably for a number of reasons. I think the main ones go about like this:

> "I won't stick with it anyway, so why embarrass myself when I quit."

> "I don't want the pressure of going to workouts just because someone else wants to go."

> "It will be easier to quit."

> "It will be easier to skip workouts."

> "My workout partner will make me look bad."

> "It's not worth the effort."

So be different. It will be easier to exercise if you get others to do it with you. Other people can motivate you to do things you might not otherwise do, which means they will help you exercise more often, longer, and harder. For example, when I decided to run that first marathon, I had been running for thirteen years, and I had covered distances of as much as 17 miles at one time. I had run races for fun, from three miles to ten. But I had done so much reading about marathons and training for them that I was concerned about being able to do all the work necessary by myself. How could I force myself, alone, to run all those runs, all those miles, and all those days? I didn't think I could, so I asked some of my running friends to do it with me. We started by training for and running a half-marathon, a nice 13.1 mile run in the beautiful countryside outside Beaverton, Oregon. We even drove out to the course a few weeks before the race to see how scenic it was, to try to convince ourselves that admiring the land, trees, barns, and all of nature in its glory would surely distract us from the long run and make the time slip by. We all bought in, did some extra running in preparation, and all of us finished the half-marathon with no complaints. We were all very proud of ourselves. Then we started the training for the full marathon. The serious stuff.

Every time one of us wanted to run, there was at least one other person to run with. There were six of us training, and since four were in he same neighborhood, four was usually the minimum during each run. During our one, weekly, long run, there were usually all six of us. Run after run, we fed off each other, and after three months of intense training after the half-marathon we did the big one, and not one of us thought we could have done it alone.

Please note: in Chapter 7 on exercise, it is emphasized that setting goals that are too aggressive is a main cause of people dropping out of a new exercise program quickly, so I don't want to give the impression that running a marathon is something I encourage people to do. Not even close. I am just trying to illustrate that it is much easier to exercise, at any level, if you get some support by getting people to do it with you. To help get you started and to help keep you going. Especially in the beginning. Even if all you start with is a short stroll through the park, around the block, or through the mall. You will be much more likely to do it and stay with it if you get people to do it with. If someone else is expecting you, it will be harder for you not to go.

You can do it, just try to do it with some friends.

12

"Doc, It Hurts When I Do This." "Then Don't Do That."

or,

The Irresponsibility of the Medical Community and Other Credentialed People and Organizations

We need to be able to rely on doctors, and I love doctors, and "some of my best friends are doctors." However, I feel a need to express a concern about some doctors I don't know, but have heard about.

It goes like this. We have a wealth of information about how our lifestyle has caused many problems, and we have the knowledge to fix those problems, but I don't believe the medical community is doing enough to make things better. Specifically, we know that Americans eat vast quantities of excess fat which often leads to weight gain and ill health, and we know that diets actually cause weight gain over time which further aggravates an already bad situation. But there are doctors who still put people on diets and who are still not being emphatic about all the fat their overweight patients eat. Doctors need to be more involved with solutions by being specific and persistent in telling their patients in no uncertain terms what caused the problems, what to do to begin making things better, and to follow up to help ensure improvement. Doctors need to take the lead.

The same can be said for many other formally trained people involved with the health, fitness, and well-being of people, such as nutritionists. Most of these continue to teach that a person can get up to 30% of their calories from fat. But 30% is too high. The U.S. government distributes the same bad advice by mandating that this 30% guideline be placed on the labels of the food we eat. We are literally surrounded with bad information, and most all of it comes from the prominent figures, professionals, and institutions that not only should know better, but that should be leading the charge to get things right. This is really bad news.

If your doctor, nutritionist, or whoever gives you bad advice like the 30% rule noted above or tells you to go on a diet, you need to find a different doctor, nutritionist, or whoever.

Note

Let me add something, for the doubters. Both the American Medical Association and the American Heart Association recommend limiting the amount of calories we get from fat to 30% of total calories. I believe that if you raise a kid on 30%, that kid will grow up to be overweight and unhealthy with elevated cholesterol and partially clogged arteries. Furthermore, the typical adult American has been getting around 40% of their calories from fat and is overweight with elevated cholesterol and partially clogged arteries. If that typical American attempts to fix those three things by reducing the amount of calories they get from fat down to the 30% recommended by all these trained, educated professionals, prestigious organizations, and the U.S. government, he or she will see little or no improvement, as far as I am concerned. Because 30% is too high. All these highly visibly and influential institutions and people should be scolded. If we can't rely on them we are in real trouble, but of course we have been and we are.

13

Excuses, Excuses, and More Excuses

In doing the research for this book, I collected a lot of information. When I had as much as I thought necessary, I reviewed the articles and other materials and marked each piece I was going to save with the appropriate chapter number. Then the items were put in folders. Some of the folders were quite full. As I prepared to write this chapter, I opened the folder marked "Chapter 13," and found just one small piece of paper, with the following:

"Excuses are endless, easy, and free."

I don't know where I got it, so my apologies to someone. But that statement says it all, and it applies to about anything. If we want to get more education, or change jobs, or learn how to play the piano, or get healthy, fit, and thin, the excuses for not doing so are endless, easy, and free.

What interests me, though, in regards to being healthy, fit, and thin, is that it would seem everyone would want to be healthy, fit, and thin, so everyone would do whatever is necessary to be like that. Especially if doing so was not difficult, which it isn't. After all, we are talking about life and our health and well-being, and looking and feeling our best. But as we know, the majority of people are overweight, unhealthy, and unfit. So what gives?

I think the answer is two-fold. First, many people probably do attempt change in regards to their eating habits, but the changes are weak, not consistent, or based on bad information that actually makes the problems worse. For these people, the issue is not excuses, but rather reality, the giving up of what doesn't work. For the rest, those who continue to make excuses, let me just say that the changes necessary are not that difficult, I promise. Once a person begins the process of eating correctly and exercising, the easier it gets. The changes become the norm.

So start, stick with it, and enjoy all the good life has to offer without the problems. You won't have to make excuses for that.

14

"It's In My Genes." "No, It's In Your Jeans."

I remember when I was in my teens checking out, with my buddies, teenage girls, and if we saw one who was not overweight but who was with her mother who was overweight, someone would usually say about the young girl, "Watch out for her. She will grow up to be fat, just like her mom." The assumption being made was that the girl's genes were what were going to make her gain weight, but we now know, we really do know, that the genes play virtually no role in obesity. The girl will become overweight like her mom if she eats like her mom.

Earlier in the book, in Chapter 2 about the consequences of eating huge amounts of excess fat, we pretty much laid this gene thing to rest, without addressing it directly. We said that you can only become overweight by improper eating, which in large part means eating excess fat, and that eliminates heredity. But, since the gene myth is so strong, it gets in the way of resolution. So, we need to deal directly with it. To end the myth.

We have seen that bad information has very negative effects on our health and well-being, and in this area of heredity the same thing holds. For example, in 1994 it was announced that a gene had been found in mice that caused mice to get fat. We then had a "fat gene." Proof. The assumption was made that this discovery would lead to the same finding in humans. It didn't matter that there was no evidence that such a gene would be found in humans. Suddenly, many over-weight people just shrugged their collective shoulders, and said, "See, it's not me, it's my genes, now pass the donuts." People took a bit of information, in this case the potential of a fat gene in mice, to explain away their obesity.

Let's look at some more ill-founded logic, from an article in the Chicago Tribune, December 11, 1994, titled "Fill 'er up." Please note that I hold nothing against the writer or the newspaper. Both are just reporting what is going on, and I love the Tribune, and start every day with it as I drink coffee out of my Chicago Tribune coffee cup. Any-way, one part says, "Genetic heritage influences individual metabolism in a way that greatly complicates even the most determined efforts many people make to lose weight and keep it off." We know genes can differ from person to person, but we also know that you can't make something out of nothing. If people spend their whole lives eating badly, they are going to become overweight, clog up their arteries, and raise their cholesterol to dangerously high levels, regardless of what their genes, or heredity, or metabolism might be. No matter what.

A Fact of Life

A pause here to take a closer look at a related issue, again. To further clarify. It was noted in Chapter 6, that as we get older our metabolism slows down. From wherever it is, it slows down, so unless a person manages their lifestyle properly, they will gain weight as they age. This applies to the entire human race, not just to certain people, and explains why most people gain weight as they age. This is not about genes the way I look at it. It is about the body's natural reaction to the aging process. There is a big difference.

Back to the article: "Studies show, for example, that many obese people eat little or not more than those whose weight stays within nor-mal range without much effort." Now, we saw earlier in this book that overweight people often eat less than thin people, so let's not use this as some mystery that needs solving by a series of long-term, comprehensive, expensive studies. Overweight people, over time, mess up their metabolism so much that even eating small quantities of food can cause additional weight gain. And that sentence states, "…than those whose weight stays within a normal range without much effort." My weight stays in a normal range with zero effort, because I eat right and exercise. I have done so for decades, and the eating right has become easy, natural, normal, and habit, while the exercise has become so easy as to be effortless. But there is even more in just this one article: "There isn't a single answer to the medical and social problems of obesity." That sounds pretty dramatic, and it is just that kind of thinking that makes matters worse. We have seen that bad eating, which in large part means eating excess fat, begets fat. So, there is a single solution for the prevention of obesity and all its health problems: eating right.

Done? Not yet. The article ends with this: "But maybe the new and increasing evidence about the biological causes of obesity will reduce a little of the guilt that society imposes on us and we on ourselves." We don't need more evidence, and we do not need to suffer guilt. We have the answers.

I don't know where the saying "don't beat a dead horse to death" comes from, but let me beat this heredity thing some more. In a report from the Medical College of Wisconsin (Chicago Tribune 11-22-94), it was announced that "a multimillion-dollar research effort to identify—and perhaps alter—the genetic roots of obesity" would be undertaken. The research project "will try to track the root causes of obesity, seeking out the gene—or genes—that may affect appetite, caloric balance and the growth of fat tissue." More proof that we must be stupid. We know what causes obesity. Genes might certainly influence the base rate at which the body burns calories, but eating excess fat and doing other bad things regarding eating habits will still cause weight gain. Period.

Our genes take tens of thousands of years to change. Or millions of years, or whatever. A real, real long time. But as a society, we became overweight almost overnight. What happened that night was that fast food/fat food places sprang up everywhere. We started eating huge amounts of french fries, cheeseburgers and pizza. Wolfing down that stuff and becoming overweight, clogging up our arteries, and sending our cholesterol through the roof. Our genes didn't change, only the size of our jeans...upward.

We know what caused the problems, and we know the solutions.

Hot Off The Press

Here I am, the book is finished, I am just doing some final editing, and today's Chicago Tribune (5-02-02) has the following article right there on the front page: "Obesity giving adult illnesses to kids." It says we have an epidemic of obesity in kids, and that the rates of such have "...doubled in the last two decades..." The genes of our kids did not change this quickly. The kids' jeans did. To a larger size. We need to stop fooling ourselves.

15

Stress (Chill Out. Relax. Life Is Real Short, Right Suzie?)

Easier said than done. Everyone is stressed out, and while it is normal to experience some degree of stress, we stress about anything and everything and wind up far more stressed than we need to be. We stress about things that didn't even exist just a short time ago. People stress because their computer is too slow, yet that computer is lightning fast compared to the computer this same person had only a few years ago, which was miraculously fast when first purchased but was stressfully slow shortly after that. And not long before this computer was bought, there wasn't even such a thing as a computer. We keep piling it on ourselves.

From an article by Bob Condor in the Chicago Tribune (10-3-01): "Research shows about 75 percent of Americans say they experience 'great stress' on a weekly basis. That's up from the 55 percent reported in the same independent study commissioned by Prevention Magazine in 1983.

"The statistics are not surprising. Americans know they are stressed out. They spend billions on potential remedies ranging from decaffeinated coffee (a $1 billion annual business) to anti-anxiety pills ($2 billion) to books and workshops ($42 billion).

"Yet the stress epidemic stays on record pace."

It's interesting that over the last 20 to 30 years as we ate worse and worse, exercised less and less, and became ever more sedentary via the dumb box (TV), we became more and more stressed out. Let's see where this all comes together, as if we don't already know.

As Condor went on to write, the issue with stress is the damage it does not just on the psychological side but also the physical. "Although we tend to think of stress as an emotional component of health, doctors and scientists are clearly finding significant and disturbing physical effects on the cardiovascular and immune systems." In this article Dr. Benjamin Fusman, a cardiologist at the University of Chicago, is quoted as saying, "People under stress experience increased blood pressure, heart rate and respiratory rate. There is also a change in the blood platelets; they tend to be more sticky, and that's when people can develop heart attacks." Condor then wrote: "Interpretation: If you lead a sedentary life, eat too much saturated fat, don't get enough sleep and subject yourself to constant stress, these risk factors can align in a dangerous fashion."

So on top of the damages we have been doing to ourselves by our bad eating habits and lack of exercise, we add the damages caused by stress. But all is not bleak. The first thing mentioned in the article regarding the effective management of stress is exercise, and that is good news, obviously, because it is part of the same remedy we are going to use to deal with our other issues. The answer is always the same.

Exercise is a phenomenal stress reliever, one which I was fortunate to have discovered thirty-two years ago. I first began running in 1970 while in the Air Force in South Korea. I was twenty-two years old in a very stressful environment, and I started exercising to deal with the stress, and it worked. I have been running ever since, and I have learned firsthand the tremendous psychological as well as physical benefits of exercise. In fact, I have said for a long time that I only run for my head, and the physical side follows. While running I relax, think, and solve problems. Tension goes away, the spirit is lifted, and I feel great. It's exhilarating, and the best stress reliever I can imagine.

This is wonderful news, wouldn't you agree? You are going to exercise anyway to help yourself become physically healthy, fit, and thin, and the exercise you are going to do is going to help you to chill out. Exercise is so good, that if I could do it more often, I might be too chilled. Frozen.

Oh, and by the way, in Mr. Condor's piece, in regards to relieving stress, Dr. Karen Koffler, director of the integrative-medicine program at Evanston Northwestern Health Care, is quoted as saying, "Watching TV doesn't cut it, even if it is sports or entertainment…" Now you have it from someone higher up the smart chart than me, turn the stupid TV off. Read a book, take it easy, relax, and go to bed earlier. A good night's sleep will dramatically help you to get frozen, I mean to chill out.

Just Ask Suzie

The title to this chapter mentions Suzie. That would be Dukes, as she is referred to by those she grew up with. Suzie Dukes, my long-time friend. Way back when she and I were in our early teens, we decided we wanted to be friends for life, so we didn't do any boyfriend/girlfriend stuff that could have caused us to separate for good. Today, nearly forty years later, we are still friends. We talk about the good old days, and celebrate them, but the point is always that time goes by quickly. That we have to also celebrate this day. We need to live the day as best we can, relish it, do something good for ourselves and someone else, and make each day important. We can only do all that if we don't get hung up on the small things. Only if we don't stress about things that are not worth worry. We need to live life, love life, and share life.

Be cool.

16

Willpower, Discipline, Motivation and SEX

"How in the heck do you expect me to get healthy, fit, and thin? I mean, hey, it has taken me my whole life to get like I am today, to where so much is wrong. Give me the secret, the magic that will get me started down the road to weight loss, healthiness, thinness, and all the rest," asked the fat guy.

In response, he was offered, for free, the solution. "OK. Here it is…the magic…the secret…a drum roll please: I hereby and herewith bequeath you with…motivation.

"Now that you have it, you will not lose it, and you will not only do all the things necessary to become healthy, fit and thin, but you will be able to do anything else you want to do. You can now write the great American novel, or become the president of a gigantic, worldwide corporation, or realize your dream of becoming a movie star. Your biggest problem now, and maybe your only problem, is to figure out what not to do, now that you have motivation."

But seriously. There is a huge market that sells motivation techniques, but I didn't do any research to discover just how big that market actually is, because I am not motivated to do so. I do know that people spend billions of dollars a year on books, videos, cassettes, and seminars to learn how to become motivated, while companies kick in more billions for the same stuff to motivate their employees. Kind of like the weight loss industry, you know, give 'em a new twist even though it also won't help, and in comes some more dough. Haven't we all had it pounded into our heads that motivation is the key? We've got to get motivated, or she succeeded because she was motivated, or he failed because he wasn't motivated enough. Get motivated. That's all there is to it.

Nonsense. You will accomplish things if you want to, and that is all there is to it. If you have had thoughts about learning how to play the piano, and you have spent years trying to muster up the motivation, but you have yet to even schedule your first lesson, not to mention taking hundreds of lessons and actually practicing thousands of hours, you do not really want to learn to play the piano. Likewise, if you are unhealthy, overweight, and unfit, you will begin the process of fixing those problems only when you want to, not when you get "motivated." If you want it, you will do it.

The same goes for willpower. The Oxford Essential Dictionary defines willpower as "control exercised by deliberate purpose over impulse." If doing what is necessary to become healthy, fit, and thin has to be so deliberate and so controlling, nothing good is going to happen.

Discipline. We can go on for a long time here, but we are going to wind up in the same place, as far as I am concerned.

I have been running for 32 years, and I continue to do so for the simple reason that I want to. Motivation, willpower, and discipline play absolutely no role in my running. I run, and the only reason I will likely continue to run for the rest of my life is because I want to. So, if you see me running, or someone else running, don't look and ponder about how I or they are doing that, how we managed to get the motivation or whatever to do that. Ponder not. We want to.

"You want to what?"

I am not a philosopher either. But for years I have been saying one consistent thing regarding the running of a marathon, and it sounds simple, because it is. The statement is: "You can't run 26.2 miles unless you want to." The amount of work, time, effort, training, and all the other things that go into the preparation and successful completion of a marathon are extensive. The planning. When to run, where, and for how long? What if you are traveling regularly for business? I remember one evening during the training for my first marathon when we had to drive to a different neighborhood to run, because it was raining so hard that we would have had trouble running our normal route. That course was partly along unpaved roads which would have been too muddy. So we drove to a residential area a few miles away, parked the car and ran five miles. It rained hard the whole way, and it was cold. When we returned to the car we were all cold and soaking wet, and then someone said, "Let's do it again." We all ran that second five miles, as difficult as it was, not because of any motivation, discipline, willpower, courage, or craziness. We ran it because we wanted to. If you want to become healthy, fit, and thin, you will do so because you want to, and doing so will be infinitely easier than training for a marathon.

"and SEX"

Oh, and about sex. That was put in the chapter title just to get your attention. I am not done researching the topic, so I can't offer any conclusive advice at this time.

See ya.

17

Drugs, Pills, Herbals, Miracles, Natural Remedies, Vitamins, Minerals, Supplements, Zen-Zen, I Mean Fen-Phen, And Other Stupid Things

Take two aspirin and call me in the morning.

Wait, I've got an even better deal. I am going to invent a pill that will do a whole lot more than aspirin. This one will not only cure your headache, it will also make you healthy, fit, and thin. Just take it with water three times a day. In only 30 days you will see amazing results. If you are a woman, you will become prettier, your hair will get nicer, you will get those thighs you've always wanted, and your breasts will become large, perfect, and just plain spectacular. You will become beautiful and sexy.

If you are a man, you will become handsome, your muscles will become large and ripply, your hair will become thick and full, and if your hair has gone away, it will grow back. Women will find you irresistible. Your biggest problem will be choosing which women you want.

When I get this pill ready for the market, how much do you think I will be able to sell it for? What will a person who is overweight and unhealthy as a result of a lifetime of bad habits, who is unhappy about their situation, who has tried endless streams of miracle health and weight-loss plans, scams and schemes year after decade only to see things get worse, pay for my pill?

Americans spend tens of billions of dollars every year on attempts at remedy, most of which don't work. The amount spent averages out to something like $192,000,000 per day. (Really. I didn't make this up. I just don't remember where I heard it. But it's real.) If they spend that on things that don't work, what would my pill be worth? Trillions? I will settle for only what people are spending now on the worthless stuff, and I will work just one more day the rest of my life. I would make well over $100 million dollars that one day, after expenses. Then some huge company would see what I have and buy me out for about $100 billion or zillion or whatever. I will be set for life, and soon everyone will be healthy, fit, and thin. I will be real happy and so will hundreds of millions of other people. I will be a hero, too, although I don't aspire to that at all. In fact, I think I will take some of my money and have surgery on my face, so I can live a normal life without sainthood.

So what will my pill be worth? I expect that some people will pay $1,000 for a 30 day supply, and some people, those who are in real bad shape and who are rich, will pay me $100,000. Maybe even $1,000,000. But wait. Are you thinking I'm crazy? There cannot ever be such a pill. Right? I guess I'm out of luck.

But wait again. There is a pill, and actually lots of pills, already on the market, that promise everything I was going to promise and even more. There goes my fortune. By the way, I was way off on the price, because where I was going to charge like tens of thousands of dollars because it seems that is what such a pill would be worth, people can actually buy a month's supply of what is already available for next to nothing. I will be sad to show you.

By now you probably know where I am going with this. You can only become healthy, fit, and thin if you eat right and exercise. There is no magic, no secret, no short cut. The reason I am writing this chapter, though, is because there are so many people who believe there are miracles. Since I want to do all I can to help people, perhaps looking at stupid things will help. If people can learn to ignore the ridiculous and identify the good, they will be better able to succeed.

Some Crazy Stuff

To help show the difference between the ridiculous and the good, I collected a lot of crazy advertisements, but there is one that is more mind-boggling in its stupidity than all the rest. A full page ad, in color, with a lot to read, and a picture of a stunning woman. She is beautiful and shapely; she has long glorious hair, a thin waist, a happy smile, the works. The headline reads: "Lose Up To 50 Pounds Without Dieting!" Reading between the lines, it says try this and look like this fine, sexy woman. Now look at the actual words, and keep in mind that all of them come from just this one ad:

> "New Medical Breakthrough!"

> "…scientists have finally developed an extra-strength, fast acting weight-loss formula that eliminates dieting, eliminates strenuous exercise, and most importantly, eliminates fat, flab, and cellulite."

> "…enhances muscle tone without exercise, so you are left with a sleek, firm, and youthful new figure."

> "…you can eat all your favorite foods and still lose weight!"

Absolutely incredible. There I was, planning on selling my magic pill for as much as $100,000 for a one day supply, and instead, you can buy a full eight-week supply of Chromolite 3® for just the small amount of $49.95, or only 89 cents per day. An eight-week supply of my magic stew would cost $5,600,000, and here a person can buy something that is already on the market, no waiting for me to invent it, for just pennies. And their pill does more than I ever thought mine would. I never dreamed that my pill would also give a person a sleek, firm, and youthful new figure.

How much more stupid can it get? Just watch.

Here's a catchy ad that shows another sexy woman, in a bikini, in the arms of a hunk (I guess) of a man on the beach. The headline here says, "Hollywood's new diet phenomenon, lose up to 10 pounds this weekend…while you cleanse, detoxify and rejuvenate your body." This ad, too, keeps getting better the more you read. For example, it goes on to say that this diet is "the faster and easier Miracle Diet," which implies that there are other miracle diets, but this miracle is better, because it is faster and easier. I didn't know that miracles could be fast or slow or easy or hard. This ad apparently is educational beyond diets. Then it goes on to say, "It's what actors, actresses and models use to fit into those sleek suits and sexy dresses—fast!" Amazing how stupid this stuff can be.

Here's an ad, with another beautiful, thin, shapely woman wearing just a bra and panties, and she is holding a pineapple. Hold on. I know what you are thinking, but you are wrong. You are thinking it's about eating pineapples to lose weight, but that is incorrect, because, as the ad points out, while it has been scientifically proven that if you eat 10 to 12 pineapples per day you will lose weight "before your very eyes," it is "impossible to eat so many pineapples per day." So, it's been done, but it can't be done, but when it is done you lose weight. Anyway, the ad then says "The amazing discovery…is that they took the magic that is in the pineapple that causes the weight loss and put it in pill form. When you then take the pills, during the entire duration of your weight loss:

> "You will never be hungry."

> "You will not be on any diet."

> "You will not have to exercise."

> "You will not have to sacrifice anything whatsoever."

The ad gets even more ridiculous, believe it or not, but it is so bad, we will move on. I have 15 more ads all promising miracles, but I will spare you. But how about this one I received, unsolicited, via the internet:

"In Thousands of Clinical Studies, GH Has Been Shown to Accomplish the Following":

> "Reduce body fat and build lean muscle WITHOUT EXERCISE!"

> "Enhance sexual performance."

> "Remove wrinkles and cellulite."

> "Lower blood pressure and improve cholesterol profile."

> "Improve sleep, vision and memory."

> "Restore hair color and growth."

> "Strengthen the immune system."

> "Increase energy and cardiac output."

> "Turn back your body's biological time clock 10-20 years in 6 months of usage!!!"

Now that really is magic. Here I sit at the age of fifty-three, I've been trying to eat right for over two decades now, I've been running for thirty-two years, and now I see that I didn't have to do any of that. I only had to take this magic pill. Excuse me a minute while I go phone in my order, and the next time you see me I'll be skinny. I will also have the highest performance rating possible for my enhanced sexual performance, my wrinkles will be gone, my blood pressure will have gone down, I'll be sleeping better, my vision and memory will have improved, the gray in my hair will have disappeared, and I will look ten to twenty years younger. I will have to wear a name tag, so those who know me will be able to recognize me.

There is a footnote to the magic pill ad just described. They are looking for sales reps! Believe me, with magic like this, word of mouth will reach all 3 billion of us quickly.

That's enough of the truly stupid. Now we will move up to things that are just bad. They aren't as stupid, because the way they are presented seems to be more realistic, but the end result is the same. I just want to review a few things that even more discerning people get caught up in.

I know personally of educated, successful, and seemingly intelligent people who take large doses of chromium picolinate. This so-called dietary supplement is popular with fitness fanatics and people who are trying to lose weight. It is among dozens of supplements that profess to do great things for the body. The reason these supplements are a step above the stupid is because there is at least a basis to build from. To the point, chromium picolinate comes from a specific and builds up to the ridiculous, like this:

> First…chromium is a nutritionally essential mineral.

> Then…as seen in an ad for chromium picolinate: "Nine confirming scientific studies with humans and animals demonstrate a significant reduction is body fat when chromium picolinate is added to the diet!"

> Therefore…since it's true that chromium picolinate is essential and has shown to cause weight loss in some un-specified studies, massive amounts will make you skinny.

Baloney. If this was true, everyone would be thin. The ad just mentioned also says the following, and we need another drum roll here, because something spectacular and profound is about to be witnessed:

"Combining it (chromium picolinate) with a lifestyle of low-fat eating and everyday exercise can improve both health and fitness."

I assure you that low-fat eating and everyday exercise will improve both a person's health and fitness, whether they take chromium picolinate or not. See how companies try to slip things past us? Of course we will be thin. Duh. We are overweight because we eat fat and don't exercise. Not because we don't take chromium picolinate. But I admire the chromium picolinate ad I am referencing here, because, yes, you guessed it; it contains a fine looking woman. If chromium picolinate can make a woman look like that…

By the way, as reported in the Chicago Tribune (10-26-95), "Chromium picolinate, a dietary supplement popular among fitness buffs and people trying to lose weight, has been shown in tests done on cells grown in the laboratory to cause severe damage to chromosomes." Add this to that: "We recently found a report of kidney damage caused by six weeks of chromium picolinate…" (The Bakersfield Californian, Joe and Theresa Graedon in their column "People's Pharmacy, 6-26-97).

Phen-fen

Phen-fen, the proven miracle, then splat. Here's a headline from the Sacramento Bee (4-19-97): "The weight is over…For many dieters, phen-fen is a dream come true…" It worked too. A lot of people lost a lot of weight. I have numerous articles touting this miracle weight loss duo. Take pills, get skinny. They were very popular, and then guess what? They turned out not to be miracles either. People started developing heart problems that could ruin a person's health and could potentially even lead to death. There are no miracles, and while we might have, in the beginning, put phen-fen further up the scale, because it had the approval of the federal government, the fact remained that instead of eating right and exercising to become healthy, fit, and thin, pills were taken, and the overall results were possibly very damaging.

There are no miracles, and there probably never will be. If there ever are, it will likely be a long way off, and based on our experience even with government approved miracles, a long period of successful testing would have to be done before the label "miracle" could be applied. So, without me being a scientist, I project that if there ever is a pill or other such wonderful, no-effort-required quick-fix that will make people healthy, fit, and thin, it will be a very long time from now, something like fifty to two hundred years. So, do the math and check the odds. You and I came along too early. We are going to just have to go back to the simplest, surest cure of all, eating right and exercising. We can do it. Before we start, though, we have to finish the stupid and the ridiculous.

Herbs

For centuries herbal remedies have been used to treat just about any physical problem people might have, and there is no doubt that a lot of benefit has been experienced. There are problems for us here, though, regarding herbs. One is the belief that "if a little works a lot is better." For example, it was reported a few years ago that the herb gingko biloba can improve the memory of people with dementia. Dementia is serious, as this definition from The Oxford Desk Dictionary and Thesaurus shows: "chronic or persistent insanity marked by memory disorders, impaired reasoning, etc., due to brain disease or injury." The leap was then made by companies selling the herb that it would improve everyone's memory. There is no evidence that I have found to support this claim, but companies and spokespeople have made tons of money promoting and selling gingko biloba with, for all practical purposes, no benefits, while holding doubt as to the safety of large doses.

The other problem is created by companies promoting the idea that anything natural must be safe and effective. In fact, they don't even hint at it, they just flat out say it, in ways such as, "It's safe and effective, because it's natural." Now, since we have been looking at stupid things, and we're therefore getting pretty good at identifying stupid things, we won't have to delve into this natural-is-safe-and-effective very deeply to see the stupidity. Watch. There are plants, that if you eat them, will not only not cure anything, but that will make you sick and some that will kill you, some almost instantly. Natural means nothing. Absolutely nothing. Of course it is true that there are natural things that can help certain conditions and still be safe in controlled quantities, but to say everything natural is safe and effective is ridiculous.

Some further clarification is in order here also, because of more intentionally misleading information. When the weight loss drugs phen-fen were taken off the market, companies started promoting what was referred to as "herbal phen-fen." This caused desperate dieters to flock to dietary supplements bearing names such as Herbal Phen-fen and Herbal Phen Fuel. We then had overweight people using herbals that were not approved or proven, in place of government approved drugs that could kill people. People switched to herbal magic, but if it was magic, why didn't we already know it so the magic would have made the real phen-fen unnecessary in the first place? The answer here is obvious also. There is no magic, and just because something is natural, or herbal, does not mean it can benefit you in any way.

Finished yet, you might ask? No, but, almost, and I will try to finish with a flare. I have the perfect ending to this chapter. A new drug. Approved even. I give you Xenical ™. From its ad in a magazine: "It's a unique prescription weight loss medication that, when combined with a good meal, can actually help you lose weight." But wait. There's more, "you may experience gas with oily discharge, increased bowel movements, an urgent need to have bowel movements and an inability to control them, particularly after meals containing more fat than recommended." Comedians could have a field day with this. Since I'm not a funny guy, I won't even attempt humor. But, think about it. An overweight person, instead of doing the simple, tried-and-true weight loss program of eating right and exercising, decides to take this magic pill. Just imagine what could happen and where. In a big, important business meeting, or in an interview for a long sought after job, or on a date with a high-potential person, when all of a sudden…

Stupid is as stupid does. There are no miracles, pills, drugs, or herbals that will make you healthy, fit, and thin, but there are a lot of such things that can harm you.

I leave this chapter on a positive note by saying that all this is more good news. Good in the sense that so many people for far too long have tried to reverse the negative effects of the good life, but to no avail. Not only have things not improved, but they have become worse. Now positive change can come about.

18

Ageless Wonders: For the Old, Older, and Oldest

I am one of you. I am 53 years old, and my knee hurts as I write this. I didn't do anything to cause the knee to hurt. I didn't fall or run into something or hurt it running. It hurts because it is 53 years old. I'm not going to a doctor, because in a few days the discomfort will go away. This is just the way it is. I am getting older. I can't physically do some of the things I used to do. If I was to drink coffee using my left hand instead of my right hand, I might pull a muscle in my left arm. I recently pulled a muscle in my back playing golf, and that is the first time in 37 years of golf that I ever got hurt playing the game. But, I am having fun getting older.

There are a lot of good things about getting older. Like not caring about what people think about the way you look, even if you look funny walking, like I do with a sore knee. The issue becomes enjoying life. The important stuff.

We Baby Boomers and older folks have accepted our age, and we are excited about the future that is upon us. But we also know that our years of living the good life have put us at an increased risk of health problems. Our long-lived lifestyles have come home to possibly interfere with our future enjoyment of life, and we want to fix whatever we can.

For most of our lives, we heard little or nothing about the harm of what now are obviously damaging activities. When we were young, many of us smoked, and except for trite remonstrations such as "that isn't good for you," or "smoking makes you smell bad," not much else was said or known. People smoked in houses they visited even if the people being visited didn't smoke. People would light cigarettes at the dining table and puff in front of a table full of people who not only didn't smoke but who were still eating. Today I think it is legal to shoot anyone who lights up in such a manner (just kidding about the shooting…another disclaimer).Remember people putting out their cigarettes in their mashed potatoes? Smokers would always leave some mashed potatoes on their plates just for this purpose. How about working out, or exercising to be healthy? Almost unheard of. I don't recall any health clubs being around in the 50's and 60's when we were growing up. Do you remember even one? Did your parents "work out?" Was your mom a runner?

How old were we the first time we heard about the evils of eating food with too much fat? We were already middle-aged. I was 15 years old when the first McDonald's came on my scene, and it was great, and not once did anyone express concern about the health issues associated with eating cheeseburgers and french fries. Around that same time I had my first pizza, at the original Shakey's® in Sacramento. That pizza remains the best I ever had, and again no mention. We started eating all kinds of extra fat and calories, not thinking the slightest thing was wrong. To some extent we can be excused, or at least could have been excused for a while, compared to young people today who should know full well the dangers of eating fat food/junk food.

One quick thing here to help emphasize the evolution of our habits, before we move on to addressing ways we can go about reversing things and getting on with enjoying our old, older, and oldest selves. Not long ago I was talking to a woman in her 30's, and she asked me, "Why weren't our grandparents fat? All they ate were meat and potatoes." I responded, "Because they didn't have Twinkies®." It is only recently that massive amounts of additional fat have come into our diets. When you look at all the extremely high-fat food we have been eating that our parents and their parents did not eat because those foods didn't even exist, some of our problems become obvious. French fries, pizza, chips and on and on. Before I go on, back to Twinkies. I love them, and I don't mean to single them out as bad, but the word just came out. I still eat a Twinkie now and then, and you can too, once you become healthy, fit, and thin.

Twinkies

When I was six years old I went to the birthday party of a kid turning six. I remember playing games, specifically musical chairs, in a fenced back yard on a beautiful, warm, clear day in Sacramento. After the games we all went inside for snacks, and I will never forget what I saw in that house some 47 years ago. On a table were piles of Hostess® products, Cup Cakes, Snow Balls, and Twinkies. I had never been so impressed with anything in my whole six-year life. Glorious, and obviously a certain sign of wealth. The good life. Now back to real life.

Back To It

Most of the old, older, and oldest of us have been eating badly for decades. They have not exercised either. Their health is at risk, but they want to enjoy their age, their life, and their success. The directions for doing so are easy as shown throughout this book. The new part here is that due to their age, they have to start now. Tomorrow won't do, because tomorrow is already here. It arrived when we weren't looking.

Specifically, the following are what must be done by us Boomers and folks who are even older. Much of what is below has been discussed earlier in the book, but I offer them again here to reinforce their importance, and to add a few things that might help instill some timeliness to your response, to get you going sooner and with more resolve:

1. Get a complete physical. (This is for every adult, regardless of age.) Tell your doctor why. "Doctor, I am now _____ years old, and I haven't taken all that good of care of myself. I have been eating badly all my life, and I have never exercised. I am not nearly in the condition I want to be, so I am going to start eating right and exercising. I want to know specifically what my medical condition is before I start exercising. I don't want to be glanced at and told that I am in good condition relative to most people my age. I want to know what my heart and my cardiovascular system are doing, if my arteries are beginning to get plugged up, and what my cholesterol level is. Help me, Doc. Take this seriously, please." If the doctor doesn't take it seriously, find a doctor who will.

2. Begin exercising as soon as your doctor says "go," by using the formula in Chapter 7. I have seen dozens, if not hundreds, of articles over the years, as you likely have, detailing how effective exercise can be for people as they get older. Start exercising, do whatever you have to do to do it regularly, build up to a consistent, effective level, and stick with it.

3. Start eating properly right this minute. (Please refer to Chapter 4.)

4. Once you have been eating right and exercising for at least 3 months, and you feel better, weigh less, and are comfortable with all these new things, slowly begin to incorporate strength training into your program. Get some weights and a basic book on strength training, or join a health club and get some instruction. Some light weight lifting will be good for you, and it will help you invigorate yourself both physically and mentally. Do the same with stretching.

Two Things

1. <u>Sense of urgency</u>

The time to start is right now. Don't treat all this as a New Year's resolution, or "I'll get started on my next birthday," or whenever. Start moving today. Walk to the phone and call to schedule your visit to the doctor for your physical, then head to the kitchen to get rid of all the junk in there, and then go to the grocery store and fill your shopping cart with good food.

2. <u>Degree of completeness</u>

You will feel better quicker, and you will help yourself to the maximum extent possible, if you do everything you can. Figure out all you need to do and do it all. Be positive about it. Come into this convinced you are going to become healthy, fit, and thin, because you now have better information than you had before. Don't go into this as a test, or as another hit or miss deal. Be positive, and don't look back.

19

Kids Are Cute…and Fat and Getting Fatter All the Time

Of course they are. Fat I mean. Maybe cute too, but certainly fat and getting fatter all the time, and it is obvious why. Their parents have lousy eating habits and the kids eat the same way as the parents. There is no mystery here either.

The fact that so many kids are overweight is bad, and it should cause alarm, and it should call for remedy. But since so many adults are in the same terrible condition and in fact keep getting worse, the kids can't be helped. This is tragic and inexcusable.

We need to help the kids. But we are going in the wrong direction, because the situation with the kids is constantly getting worse. However many are overweight today, an even higher percentage will be overweight tomorrow. The way things are going, there is no end, until of course, every kid is overweight, unhealthy and unfit. Stupid beyond words.

I have read where a lot of younger teenage girls have made it known that they would rather be dead than fat, but as many of them will see, they will get fat anyway, in spite of their passion against it. These girls, these kids, are actually helpless, because the adults are feeding them fat and bad information. On top of that these youngsters are establishing eating habits that will insure long term weight gain for virtually all of them and obesity for many.

123

From Time Magazine (1-21-2002): "…the percentage of youngsters ages 6 to 11 who are overweight has tripled since the 1960s…and doctors are seeing dangerously obese children as young as age two."

It gets worse, as the article continues. "Overweight children are more than twice as likely to have high blood pressure or heart disease as children of normal weight. Even more alarming is the number of children with Type 2, or non-insulin-dependent, diabetes. Once known as adult-onset diabetes—before so many children started getting it—Type 2 diabetes puts kids at risk for very adult ailments, including blindness, nerve damage, kidney failure and cardiovascular disease."

The Solution?

It should be obvious, but it seems to be impossible. The solution is to eat right and exercise, but the parents aren't so the kids aren't. End of story I guess. What can I offer? Everything we see about this problem talks about kids watching too much TV, but, again, so do the parents. It certainly won't work for good ol' mom and dad to tell the kids to turn off their TV only to have mom and dad return to their TV. And just sit there and eat junk.

There is only one solution, and that is for the parents to eat right, exercise, leave the TV off, and get the kids on the same program. I hope this doesn't come across as a cop out on my part, but gee whiz.

20

The Author and the DeSoto

"Are you still skinny?" The question came from Mike Reynolds, my friend from long ago. We hadn't seen each other in thirty-six years, since we were seventeen. We hadn't kept in touch, either, but through a mutual friend, Dukes as a matter of fact, we were about to get together. We were on the phone coordinating. Mike in Gridley, California, and me in Chicago.

Way back, when Mike and I last saw each other, I was skinny. I am thin today at age fifty-three. But the answer to the question wasn't "Yes, I'm still skinny." It was "I'm thin again." Unfortunately for me, along the way after age seventeen, the good life had taken over. Just like it does to most everyone. I had gone from skinny to fat, then learned and did and became thin again. Things change. (I'm using the terms skinny and thin, because there is a difference. Skinny is the absolutely-no-excess-weight thing. You know, "just skin and bones." Thin is heavier than that. At or below ideal weight, but more than skin and bones. It's hard to be skinny these days, but I'll get there again. Maybe.)

Gridley is a small town of but a few thousand people, sixty miles north of Sacramento, in the great Central Valley of California. Peaches and plums all over the place. Everyone called the plums prunes though. A prune is a dried plum, but most of the plums around Gridley were turned into prunes. So they were prunes to everyone, even when they were still on the tree, long before picking and drying. To the best of my recollection, picking-up prunes was the first real job I ever had. I was eleven years old, and I rode my bike four miles north of town to work, with my brother and one or two other guys, I don't remember who. Anyway, the prunes weren't picked from the tree. First, a piece of farm equipment shook the prunes off the tree. Then people crawled around on their hands and knees picking them up, put them in buckets, and then carried the buckets to where the boxes were. The knees began to hurt, and when you are eleven, the novelty wears off in a hurry. We were just working for Coke™ and Twinkie money, so our tenure in that orchard was short. There might be more about prunes later.

I moved to Gridley from Sacramento at age ten and remained there until age fifteen, at which time my family returned to Sacramento. When I got to Gridley I was skinny and my parents had a DeSoto. Both of those things would change. (OK you youngsters: a DeSoto was a car made by Chrysler.)

This chapter isn't about me or the DeSoto. It's about nothing. And change. However, the histories of both myself and the DeSoto started when I was five years old. That is about as far back as my memory goes. I must have been born five. From five until ten, all I did was move around outside, every minute I could, barefooted as often as possible. We lived in a small house on a street with all small houses as far as the eye could see or a kid could perceive. The lawns had clover, and bees love clover. One day a bee stung me, it hurt, and the foot swelled up. When enough days passed to where I could run around outside again, some caution was taken for a while. A short while. Just as the foot healed, my brother Larry and I were at our Aunt Doris and Uncle Bud's house playing with our cousins. Little girls. We were in their garage on a hot summer day because it was cool in there. I spotted a heavy, iron car jack resting against a wall, just asking to be lifted. So I could show off. Over my head. Dumb, but at nine years old, what else was I going to do. Then my cousin Marsha, age six, tried it and dropped it on my bare toe.

Later that summer I was running through a fig orchard. My dad would manage the harvest, and being too young to work, Larry and I just played all day. The orchard had large, dry dirt clods, and I ran into one. Barefooted and hit toe first. The same toe the jack was dropped on. I hadn't gone to the doctor after the drop, because it had been determined by my mom and Aunt Doris that it wasn't broken. But it felt like it, and now the dirt clod. I changed to shoes, and other things changed too, over time.

Run, play, roller-skate, and pull Larry in the wagons dad made. (Dad loved working with wood. I have a desk, a cedar chest, and a still perfectly round rolling pin he made when he was in high school. The wagons he made were wood and the best wagons around. He had made us two, a big one and a little one. A generation later he made another wooden wagon for my two children, sweet Stacey and sweet Jenifer.) I think I was more active than any kid other than Tom Sawyer (I just finished re-reading Tom, so he is fresh on my mind.)

When DeSotos were around there was practically no such thing as fast food and not much junk food either. The combination of movement and no fast food or junk food made for a skinny kid. Those Twinkies I had at that kid's sixth birthday party were an exception. I almost never had such treats, because our family couldn't afford them. I didn't miss them though, because life was great. I thought our family had just about everything. My dad was big on ice cream, and he managed that often enough to make us all happy. He bought the big, 3-gallon tubs and kept them in the freezer in the garage. They were too big to fit in the refrigerator in the house.

A DeSoto was all we wanted or needed too. It was a tank-like looking car. Large, bulky, and plain, with brown paint that was close to the color of rust. It overheated in the mountains. No radio, no power locks or power anything, and no air conditioning. A three-speed, manual transmission with the shifter on the steering column. One day when I was seven years old, I was with my sweet sister Pam (I have been surrounded by sweet females all my life), who was ten at the time, and we were outside walking from the front of the house to the back. We were passing the garage door and the DeSoto was parked in the driveway.

The car was so close to the door that we had to walk single file and squeeze to get between the car and the garage. Pam went first, and once I was a few feet past the car, I saw blood hit the ground. It was running down the back of Pam's leg. Then I saw the long deep cut, from the DeSoto's license plate. Time moves on and a few years later the DeSoto went away. Pam still has the scar. She is a magnificent person and the best sister in the world. Since she is older than me, that scar has been around a long time.

Life without change would not be worth diddly. Too much of the change is forced on us, though, and is bad. We need to be the ones forcing, and forcing good change. I went from skinny to fat to thin, and the DeSoto came and went. The car history was predictable, and apparently the effects of the good life are too. Live it and pay the consequences.

Since all I wanted to do was to be outside moving, and I had ice cream, life was all it could be. Tremendous. Dad sometimes brought home root beer and made root beer floats. And he made the best popcorn in the world. Things kept getting better. Then when I was ten years old, my family made that move to Gridley. Good, bad, and otherwise. I'll hit on a good or so.

I believe I threw a baseball more than any kid in history. I had a dog too, Friskie, mostly cocker spaniel, gold in color. We lived at the edge of town, the last house, so endless hours were spent walking around the fields with the dog. There was a basket put up in our driveway, so a ball was bounced and shots were taken for hundreds of hours. I had a bike which was ridden for more hours, and a paper route. The moving around was constant. Early one morning at age twelve, I was on my bike delivering the newspaper, and just as I passed the house my friend Joe Castro lived in, out flew Joe with a bunch of raw eggs. He got me twice in the back.

I was about done with my route at the time the eggs came flying, so I was home changing clothes in no time. Then off to school with an egg in each front pocket. Joe was out on the playground with his back to me. I missed with both eggs. I think I choked.

I pitched in Little League, but I wasn't very good. During the summer of age twelve my family went camping and trout fishing in the Sierras. One day during that trip I finally learned how to throw. My dad knew a lot about baseball. I didn't take my glove or a ball camping, so dad worked with rocks. It only took five rocks total. Dad said, "You need to change the way you throw. You have been throwing with your arm bent. Like this." And he threw a rock. Then he said, "Throw like this instead," and there went his second rock. It took me three rocks to get it. Home to Gridley. The next time I pitched the ball was smoking. My dad was the umpire behind the plate, and he called a fair game, as I will now prove. I had one strike to get to end the game. Even though my dad had always told me never to throw a curve, even while just playing catch, because he thought doing so could cause too much stress on a young arm, I threw one. It was beautiful. I throw right-handed and the batter was hitting right-handed, and the ball started high and inside. The kid thought it was coming at him so he jerked back. Then the ball started moving and cut down and across the middle of the strike zone. It was perfect, and my dad called it a ball. I hollered at him and people in the small crowd laughed. Since dad didn't allow me to throw a curve, he saw the ball start off high and inside and made up his mind right away. He didn't expect a curve so he didn't wait for it to curve. The next pitch was the same. I figured dad would get it right this time. "Strike three!" he yelled, loudly enough to redeem himself, and the game was over.

During that summer I learned something in addition to pitching. One evening my dad suggested I go to bed early, because we were going to be getting up early the next morning. And so it was. At 5 a.m. he got me up, fixed me a bowl of cereal, and drove me to a peach orchard. By 6 a.m., as the first light shown, I was up a tall ladder picking peaches. Dad left me with a sandwich and said he would be back to get me when I had picked two bins of peaches. Two tons, four thousand pounds. Peach fuzz all over the place, 100 degrees in the shade, and exhaustion. That is the day I switched forever from baths to showers. When I got home I tried to take a bath. With all that had gone on that day, there was a layer of dirt and peach fuzz floating on top of the bath water. When I stood up to get out of the tub, that stuff stuck to me all over, from neck to feet. I turned on the shower.

The playing, the movement, baseball, and now work, all kept me skinny. Back to Sacramento at age fifteen, and still nothing but movement. Mostly basketball. We lived across the street from an elementary school with basketball courts outside, so I probably racked up something like 954 hours each year of dribbling, shooting, and playing.

After the roughest of stabs at college, I joined the Air Force. I have pictures of me in Korea in 1970 at age twenty-two, and I was as skinny as a person could be. I played a lot of basketball in the evenings. Mostly pick-up games, three on three. Also, I played at lot of one on one with Charles Mason, a man I worked with who was ten years older than me, stronger than I was, and who hated to lose. We would often take a long lunch and go to the gym (an old airplane hangar) and beat each other half to death for an hour or so. Great stress relief. It was during this time in Korea that I started running. Still no junk food, just "three squares." Extreme movement, but the whole Korea thing was a lousy way to spend a year. My first daughter, Stacey, was only three weeks old when I left for Korea.

Then life got good again. Transferred back to the states, I settled in to domestic life. The food was a lot better and there were donuts. In the evenings, after a large home-cooked meal, sitting in front of the TV and eating nachos became the norm. (See, we all go through that TV thing. I hope I didn't suggest earlier that I was above it. The good life gets us all.) Sometimes beer and ice cream added. Really. Play and movement stopped too, except for the running, thank goodness. The running kept me from exploding. It certainly kept the pace of the weight gain down, but since we saw earlier that you "can't run it off," I couldn't run it off. The weight came. By the time I hit thirty, I was fat.

I remember the morning I stood on the bathroom scale and faced the truth. I was living in Ukiah, California, and the day before, my wife and I and two other couples had driven to San Francisco to see a 49ers/ Bears game. Junk food there, then to a Mexican restaurant for more stuffage. Then the scale. Change was in order. That was in 1980.

If I ate today the way I did when I was a young adult, I would literally weigh five hundred pounds. But the scale started me on the straight and narrow. I learned, did, and changed, but gradually. I hereby and herewith recommend that you do it suddenly, completely, and quickly. Make it easy on yourself. Recently, my great new wife Nancy and I were out for dinner. It was prime rib night at one of our favorite restaurants, and the menu offered two cuts, fourteen ounces and twenty. About halfway through our dinner a man and a woman came in and were seated at a table near us. They were around fifty years old, and the woman weighed two hundred and fifty pounds minimum, maybe three hundred. She could barely squeeze into the chair, because the chair had arms. When her meal was served, I almost fell out of my chair. She had ordered the prime rib, large. I said to Nancy, "She didn't even order the small cut." The fat lady needs to change.

I'm told change is hard, that people don't change. I have looked around, and I guess it's true, but I'm not sure it should be. Why not do things differently? Move somewhere else, change jobs or careers, go back to school, join something, do something. Learn how to play the piano or the guitar, or take cooking lessons. Use the mind. Go peach picking. So change is almost impossible? You can do whatever you want. You want to enjoy life, but things are beginning to get stacked against you. All you have to do is to begin to eat right and exercise. More change will follow. Eating right is easy, and so is exercising. If there is even one tiny hard part about exercise, it is the first step. After that it is exhilarating. Once in my life I was not able to take that first step. Maybe twice, but I can only remember the details of one. When I walked out the front door onto the porch, everything was covered with ice. It was late so there was no one to run with, and I was tired. I went back in the house.

Movement is just such a wonderful thing. It clears the mind and soothes the body and the soul. As I get older, the desire and the need to move become even greater, because it means life. I have to move.

Would you believe the more you move the more you will want to move? I don't run fast, because the act of movement is too special to ruin. Twice in my life I tried to run fast, and both times I hated it. All the relaxing, thinking, and dreaming ended with speed. When I write about the need to begin your exercise program by moving slowly, that may be all there ever is. If the first time you exercise you do it slowly and easily, and you don't do it so long that you get stressed, physically or mentally, you will feel like a queen or a king, or whatever, when you stop. You will be on your way.

You might have heard of the term "runner's high." The term refers to a feeling of euphoria that runners occasionally experience. There really is such a thing. Evidently the feeling has a physical basis. Certain duration and intensity of exercise can cause chemicals to be released into the brain that cause the feeling. I have felt it during long, easy runs, but I would not run two feet for it. I would never seek it out, because every run is good. Like sex. There are rare times, almost never, when the running can be hard, but even on these almost-never-days the bad doesn't last. I just slow down, and after twenty minutes or so the good comes back. By the time such a run is over, I wish it wasn't, just like all the rest. Then I walk. After every run, I walk. If time allows. I just want to keep moving, and you will feel this too. I promise.

We put the "I don't have time" to rest earlier in this book. The answer was turning the TV off. It doesn't seem possible that the typical adult watches 1,000 hours a year, but less than three hours a day will do it. Let's say you just cut that in half, and use those 500 hours to run. In just five years you will lose 425 pounds. Just kidding, because at some point the calories in/calories out formula doesn't work, as we saw earlier. But the plan is so simple. Move. Finding the time is really,

really easy. But I will now give you and everyone and even me the benefit of the doubt: we all need a little itty bitty bit of TV. For example, I was driving to see my grandson a couple summers ago and listening to the Cubs game on the radio. Kerry Wood was pitching and striking out batters at a record pace. I got to my grandson's in the eighth inning, turned on the TV, and told Clayton, "Come and watch this. If this keeps going like it has been, we are going to see something special. Then when you get old like me, you can tell people you saw it. With Grampy." Sure enough, Wood finished with twenty strikeouts, tying an all-time major league record. We got to see it. Yesterday I watched Tiger win the Masters, again. Other than that, life is far too short.

I started to write about changes I have made. Right here in the space you are looking at right now. But this isn't about me. However, I run slowly, and I'm not super skinny anyway, just thin. These last two years of not just the good life but the extra-good life has made it hard to be extra good. Courting Nancy and marrying her. (OK youngsters, again. Courting is dating and stuff.) Just last night we had a fine dinner at Spago. When I go to a place like that, I don't hold back. The food is just too good. So, I need to lose a few pounds. But I just got back from running forty minutes. And I won't tell you about living in Dallas with a very good job and chucking it, moving to Chicago, taking a twenty percent pay cut and not having the new job work out. Not all change turns out well, but it sure was worth a try. Changes like that Dallas to Chicago thing are a lot harder than changing to proper eating and beginning an exercise program. A bazillion times harder. Changing to feeling great is a non-event in comparison.

Do you ever hesitate to say something, because you are afraid it might sound stupid? That you will expose yourself as the only person in the world that doesn't have a firm grip on the issue at hand? Like me now, but I can stand to be embarrassed since you aren't looking at me. You can't see me blush. So here goes. I don't want to get old and regret. Sitting there stunned at age eighty with nothing on my mind other than what I could have done, should have done, and wanted to do but didn't. It seems the anguish would be unbearable. I'm thinking now, at age fifty-three, that maybe the aging process protects us from such agony. But since I am too embarrassed to ask anyone whether it does or not, I am going to make sure I do whatever I can to avoid such mental angst. Change. So I won't anguish. That explains at least one thing: why ink is hitting paper at this very moment. Along with the ink is my thought for you. Change is easy, fun, and stimulating. It only requires that first step.

That First Step, Popcorn, et al.

Maybe change is only hard because we think it is hard. How am I ever going to learn to play the guitar? I'm too old to learn, and I don't have any musical ability anyway. The answer is simple. Take lessons and practice. How are you going to start exercising? By just taking that first simple step. It's that easy. Don't over-think it. Just move. Now let's see Tom, the guy who made that first step unnecessarily difficult.

Tom ran at the rec center where I used to run. He ran five days every week, six miles each time. Fast miles too, especially for a fifty-eight year old. He told me how he started. When he was thirty-five he was tremendously overweight and a health risk at every turn. The good life. His doctor told him he was in deep trouble unless he changed everything immediately. So Tom did. But he made the first step too hard. The first time he exercised after the doctor's words, he drove to a health club, parked the car, got out of the car, leaned on the car, looked at the building, and cried. But he never looked back. I was writing at the rec center one day and I hollered as he ran by and asked, "When will your last run be," and he answered, "The day I die." He is never going to stop. It's that easy. Change is.

There is a trick to making perfect popcorn. Start by putting oil and popcorn in a pot. Just one layer of popcorn, and room for what you do put in to move around. Place the pot on the stove warmed up to the highest temperature. Gently move the pot around so the kernels and the oil heat evenly. As they begin getting hot, move the pot even faster to prevent burning. When the popcorn begins popping, put a lid on the pot, turn the stove down to medium, and raise the pot off the stove an inch or two. Keep moving it. The oil and popcorn have become as hot as you want. The popcorn will pop fast and furious. Eating right and exercising are just as easy to get right. Enjoy your popcorn.

I still enjoy prunes too. I used to make them. But first, apricots, pears, and peaches. The prunes might not mean much alone.

When I finished my last year of high school in 1966, I wanted to do something different, so I left home for the summer. Change, you know? I followed the fruit tramps around northern California, working the harvests while sleeping in barns and bunkhouses and taking baths in irrigation ditches. The first stop was to an apricot farm with Steve Watson, a friend from Gridley. Except for us two, the entire crew, not counting the foreman who was a fine Mexican fellow, consisted of broken down winos. They were men who were worn-out alcoholics with just enough left to do some work now and then, if they could stay off the hooch. In the beginning of the harvest the guys pooled their resources for a gallon of rotgut wine and put the jug in the middle of the orchard under an empty apricot box. They took turns strolling for a pull. Productivity started slipping, though, so one afternoon the man who owned the farm went storming around smashing every bottle he could find. Productivity went back up.

There was one old guy named Roy, called lyin' Roy. Always full of boloney, and his claim to fame was having been drunk 52 straight years. So he was getting desperate. Steve and I took pity on him and bought him some wine, after much pleading on his part. We drove him to the country store where he picked up a gallon. The next day Steve and I asked the Mexican foreman if we could go to his house for a Mexican dinner some time. At the end of work that same day, Juan jumped in the back seat of Steve's car and said, "Vamanos." We tried to tell him that we wanted him to first check with his wife, but he either didn't understand or he knew it would be OK. A short drive later we were at his house. It was in the middle of an apricot orchard.

An old shack with all the windows busted out. But it worked well for his summer home. In the kitchen was a fifty pound bag of tortilla flour leaning against the stove. He asked his wife to start cooking, and then he took Steve and I to the front porch to relax.

On the way to his place Juan had made us stop at the country store again, where he ran in and bought three six-packs of beer. The relaxing on the porch waiting for dinner revolved around the three of us and four of Juan's Mexican buddies drinking beer and talking. Except none of them spoke English, and we knew but a few words of Spanish. I was only seventeen, I had spent the day in the hot sun picking apricots, and I wasn't used to drinking beer, wine, or any such thing. Steve was in the same boat, and still a youngster at eighteen. Every so often Juan would check my beer and Steve's to see if we were ready for another one. If we were, he would grab the first kid running by, and it seemed like there were a dozen of them, and have them get us a fresh beer. By the time we were done with a great meal, Steve and I had each finished our six-pack and we were about shot. When we got back to the farm, we went to see old Roy, dirty bunk house and all. Steve and I slept in a barn rather than the bunk house, because the bunk house was so filthy and rundown. As tough as Steve and I might have thought we were with our summer of adventure, the bunk house was so bad we couldn't even walk in, not even one step. But with six beers apiece, we ventured in to see Roy. To our surprise, he hadn't even opened that gallon of wine. I think that if it was opened he would have had to share it with the guys, so he was still trying to figure out a way to keep it all to himself. With us as guests, he opened it. Steve and I both got sick that night.

The whole summer was about change. Doing something different. In the late afternoon prior to the final day of work, Steve and I were in the barn taking it easy. The owner, Mr. Smith, came in and asked us if we wanted to go on a plane ride. A bit of puzzlement hit Steve and me, since we were surrounded by orchards and there was certainly no real-life runway and no sign of an airplane. We said yes anyway. Neither of us had ever been on a plane. We followed Mr. Smith to a metal building near the barn. We had never given any thought to that building holding anything other than farm equipment. But that was where the plane was kept. An old, single engine prop job. The three of us pulled it out and got in. The owner started it up, warmed it up, and all the while Steve and I were without a clue as to how that thing was going to take off. But it did. All it needed was the dirt road between the trees and the irrigation ditch, and off we went, dust flying everywhere. The plane was so noisy we could only communicate with each other by screaming and so rickety we could see the ground through holes in the floor. We flew west over the foothills into a valley near the coast. When we landed, our pilot friend told us to stay in the plane, as he would just be a minute. He was delivering a box of apricots in exchange for enough fresh salmon caught that day in the ocean to feed all us fruit tramps at a barbecue the next day. The swap was quick, and off we went. As we flew back towards the farm, darkness settled in, and I hollered out the question, "How are you going to land in the dark?" I was told to look down at the irrigation ditch that ran through the farm. The moon was bright, and its reflection off the calm water lit the ditch like daylight. The pilot then shouted, "We'll land ten feet on the other side of the ditch." Right on the dirt road we had taken off from. Smooth as silk.

Don't worry about change. Good things will happen. Maybe. If not, life is surely worth continuing to try. So try again. Don't stop.

I'll skip the pear picking and the pear farmer's fine looking fifteen year old daughter and their pear-shaped swimming pool. That job didn't last long, with ten hours in the orchard and socializing every evening. Steve didn't go with me on that leg of the summer, but Lonnie Thompson, my neighborhood friend from Sacramento, did. At the pear farm Lonnie felt overworked and neglected, so after just two weeks we had to get out of there. We headed eighty miles north to the Gridley area to pick peaches. At least the pear place had showers. After the first day of picking peaches, I drove us to a nice, clean, refreshing irrigation ditch, where upon I stripped down to my shorts and jumped in with a bar of soap. After Lonnie asked what I was doing, he did it too, but he wasn't crazy about taking a bath in a ditch. At the end of the third day of peach fuzz, hard work, and 100 degree heat, Lonnie said to me, "Take me to the bus station. I'm going to go join the army. You can have all the money I've got coming. Just get me out of here."

Not long after that I went to work at a prune dryer making prunes out of plums. Thirty-two straight days, 6 a.m. to 6 p.m., tending the ovens. After work I would drive the four miles to Gridley, where friends let me shower, then to a restaurant for dinner, then back to the prune dryer for the night. I slept in the office, which was so small that a desk and soda machine took up most of the space. There was only enough room left for me to set up a portable cot. The first night there I was laying down trying to find something to listen to on the radio. It was late, dark, and not really scary, only a little. My radio was the size of two hardcover books put side by size, so it was handy to set on my chest when I was stretched out on my back in bed. It was mostly for Giant's games. Willie Mays and the guys. I was tired and half asleep when I found a station and was startled to the bone. I had found Wolf Man Jack. The Wolf Man was a famous radio DJ who made a name for himself, for among other things, loudly howling like a wolf. I had not only never heard of him, I had never heard the howl. So when my tired serenity was wracked by the clear, loud, totally unsuspected roar, I jerked wide awake. And became scared. I got up and locked the door. It took a while to get to sleep that night.

There was a nice old man, Bill, like sixty-five or so, who tended the drying of the prunes from 6 p.m. until 6 a.m. As a stupid trick, I decided to scare him, but I nearly wound up a prune myself. There were eighteen ovens, they operated at 200 degrees, and they were huge. Seven feet wide and forty feet long. The prunes were washed and spread one deep across wooden racks. Twenty racks were stacked on top of each other all riding atop a steel frame on wheels. These high stacks of prunes were moved along rails, just like railroad rails, only smaller. (As a note, my brother Larry moved the stacks from where they were put together to the front of the ovens. He had a small steel frame on wheels with a little engine attached to it. He would hook it to the stacks and move them. One day a man came to visit the farmer who owned the prune dryer. This visitor had a brand new, shinny pick-up truck. He parked close to the rails Larry went along hundreds of times a day but far enough away to not have the truck get hit. Except the pick-up truck man left the door open. Larry buckled it, and I almost died laughing. The truck man was mad, but Larry, even at the young age of 16, never hesitated to straighten someone out. "You park on the tracks; your truck gets run over." Or something like that.) A stack of fresh prunes would be moved in front of an oven. The oven would be shut off, two wide doors would be opened, and the stack rolled in. The doors were then closed and the heat turned back on. This process was repeated every ninety minutes. To make room for each new stack, a stack of finished prunes was taken out from the back end of the oven. Each drier held twelve stacks, so by moving one spot every ninety minutes, it took eighteen hours to turn plums into prunes. Physically moving the stacks through the dryer was an issue. Even though a stack weighed over six hundred pounds, it was easy enough to roll one along the rails by just pushing on it. The problem was moving eleven stacks, like this. When the oven was shut off and one stack was removed from the back of the oven, the remaining eleven stacks in the oven had to be moved back three feet to make room for the new stack. That could be done in two different ways, mine and the old guy's. But at the time I was planning to scare Bill, I didn't know there were two ways. I didn't realize he did it differently from the way I did it, until it was forced on me.

One night after returning to the dryer from dinner and noticing that Bill hadn't seen me arrive, my plan went into action. It called for me to hide near the ovens, and then once he shut off the heat and the fan for a stack change, opened the doors of an oven, and walked to the back to pull out the finished stack, I would sneak in the oven he had opened, and scare him when he came back around. So there I was, in the oven, about to jump out when all of a sudden he started to close the doors! In one split second I discovered not only that he didn't move those eleven stacks back the way I did, but I learned how he moved them. He was going to close the doors, hit the button that turned the heat and fan on, and have the power of the wind from the fan move all the stacks back. I thought I was done. It's fascinating all that can run through the mind in a fraction of a second. First, I realized that the doors closing was happening so unexpectedly and quickly that I wasn't going to be able stop them. Then I became aware that Bill was going to use the fan to move the racks back. Then I thought, wait, maybe he forgot that he had not yet put a new stack in and was going to turn the oven back on until the next cycle, ninety minutes later, at which time I would have become a crispy critter. Then I analyzed what would happen if he did, in fact, remember that he had yet to put in a new stack and was going to turn the oven and fan on just long enough to move the eleven stacks. Then I tried to determine two things from that: how long would it take and what would happen to me during that time. Finally, it was ascertained that regardless of any of the prior flashes through the head in the previous half-second or so, I better bang on the doors. I hammered as hard as I could. Just as his finger was approaching the "on" button, he heard me.

It's been great, the good life. A lot of bright spots. Wonderful people and plenty of good things. My share of bad too, but I am not suggesting more bad than average. I don't know. I'm not comparing, but at the age of fifty-three, I am thinking. I have said that however good the first fifty years were, the second will be better. Better because I am going to try harder to relish life, and that won't focus on material things like nicer cars or better steaks and finer wine. It will mean paying more attention to the way leaves grow and to the touch of the breeze on my face. The feel of life as it moves. There is no end to the real good things. All this is why I turned the TV off. To love. Life and the new wife. Whatever it is that today holds, and tomorrow, hope can only be realized if all is put into perspective. The foundation is health, our physical and mental well-being. We need to attend to us so we can attend to life and to others. One more time then: It can be easy. Please don't make it hard. And enjoy.

0-595-23396-1